Some Light at the End

Published in partnership with Works Progress Agency.
Interior & Cover Design by: Design for Writers and Studio HMVD
Illustrations by: Violet Mae Reed

A CIP record for this book is available from the Library of Congress
Cataloging-in-Publication Data.

ISBN: 978-1-7336909-7-3

An End of Life Guidebook
for Patients and Their Caregivers

Some

Light

at the **End**

By Beth Cavenaugh, RN, BSN, CHPN

Table

Introduction 1
Hospice Basics.................................... 9
Opting Out 21
Choosing Hospice................................ 29
Choices 43
Your Care 51
Visitors.. 63
Energy & Mobility 71
Eating & Drinking.............................. 91
Managing Your Medications................... 101
Pain.. 115
Constipation 131

Anxiety 139

Shortness of Breath 147

Nausea & Vomiting 157

Confusion & Delirium.............................. 165

Emergency Room Visits............................173

Processing.......................................181

As You Are Dying.................................. 197

Care for the Dying................................. 207

Acknowledgments 223

Disclaimer....................................... 227

Works Referenced................................. 229

of Contents

Introduction

Hospice is the spiritual, emotional, and physical care of
a human being at the end of their life. It is a privilege to
be a hospice nurse—I get to see the best of humanity
at a powerful time. I have witnessed deep love and honesty in
relationships, families singing at the bedside, spiritual reckon-
ings, much laughter, and messy tears. This can also be a time of
great vulnerability because it's unchartered territory; you have
never done this before. I wrote this book specifically for patients
who have just been diagnosed with a terminal illness. I want
to provide you with some guidance, support, and information
about what to expect and how to make thoughtful decisions
about your care.

I was initially exposed to end-of-life care when my mom stopped
chemo, signed up with hospice, and asked me to be her caregiver.
My son, Jack, and I moved into my parents' home for the last
three months of her life. At age one, Jack didn't have a lot to offer,
except that he delightfully distracted my mom from her lung
cancer. I didn't have a lot to offer either, frankly. I was pregnant
with my second child, tired, and unraveled. As a new nurse, this
was my first step into the world of hospice, and I didn't know
how to best help my mom.

I now have 20 years of nursing experience with over a decade's
worth of hospice. I have walked alongside many, many patients,
providing them with medical care and practical information
while supporting them emotionally at the end of their life. With
this support, patients can ease into the end of their life with more
trust and clarity. Looking back to when my mom was dying, we

had hospice support, but we were so clueless we didn't even know what questions to ask. We could have used more guidance to help us understand this process, be better informed, and anticipate the unknown.

If you're a patient who has just received a terminal diagnosis, you can still make decisions about your care, your life, and your death. I wish to reveal, with tenderness and transparency, what hospice can be in its best form so you can advocate for what you need and want. Even if you don't choose hospice, you may benefit from the information here. I will walk you through what it is like to decline and eventually die, hoping to dissolve some of the mystery and shed some light at the end. When you know what to expect, you can make informed choices about everything: your caregivers, your relationships, your medications, and even your breakfast—ice cream sundae please!

At some point you will have family, friends, or professionals involved in your care. I have thought of them every step of the way, knowing they too can benefit from basic symptom management guidance, caregiving suggestions, and the dying process. When you are tired of searching for answers under the light blue glow of the internet or you are just plain exhausted, your caregivers can use this guidebook to help you. I have chosen to include some activities and meditations designed to encourage emotional care and connection to yourself and loved ones during this time.

My hope is that you can exit this world knowing you will be taken care of and your wishes will be respected. This is your journey—I want to honor you with candor and compassion. I want you to feel cared for, to be comfortable, and to have the empowerment you deserve in this final stage of your beautiful life.

When I worked as a hospice consultant, I would visit patients to explain the benefits of hospice care. One afternoon, I walked into Jenny's hospital room. She was surrounded by her husband and three grown children, all of whom were shocked by her recent decline. I asked Jenny, "How are you?" She said, "I'm tired. I haven't slept in days because of my pain. I've been fighting cancer for two years and I can't do this anymore." We discussed her fatigue and I gently told her, "You can have a hospice nurse visit you at home three times a week, and a Home Health Aide can assist with your shower and light housekeeping a few times a week. You and your family can call us anytime day or night with any concerns."

Her disheveled husband looked slightly relieved. We talked about her pain and nausea and how hospice support may be able to assist her further. She said, "Let me think about it. Come back tomorrow."

When I walked into her hospital room the next day, she was sitting next to the window, dressed, with her hair nicely combed. She said, "I slept so well last night. I feel great. My daughter researched a clinical trial that I hope to pursue. I'm not interested in hospice." As I said my goodbyes and gave her a hug, she had a smile on her face and said, "It was lovely meeting you, but I hope the next time I see you is in the vegetable aisle at the grocery store."

I will admit I am a fan of hospice. Over the years, patients and families have shared their relief and gratitude for this support. But I'm sharing Jenny's story with you because I know hospice isn't always the right choice for everyone or it may not be the right time. Or perhaps you don't even know the questions to ask or the options available to you. Whether or not you choose hospice, I want this book to offer information that will help you make the right decisions for you.

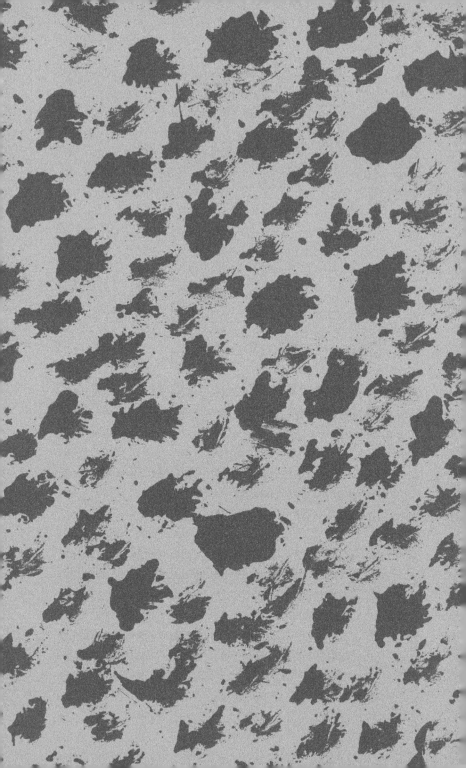

Take a
moment.

Breathe.

Hospice

Basics

Chapter 1:

Hospice Basics

When a patient hears the words, "We have done everything we can...," or "Now is the time for hospice...," most people cannot breathe, let alone think clearly, ask critical follow up questions, get support, do some research, and weigh the pros and cons. You may have been wondering how you were going to stumble out of the doctor's office safely, let alone get into a car. Or maybe you were driving on the freeway like my friend when she was told she had breast cancer. She had to pull into the hardware store parking lot to breathe. Take the time you need to center yourself.

If a physician said that you may benefit from hospice support, now is the time to gather information, clarify, and make some decisions about your care and your life. The doctors generally don't throw out the H word (hospice), unless there is a significant change in your health and you are declining, so if you are unclear, let's get some answers. Schedule another doctor's appointment or phone call once you have had a good night's rest and when you are in a more grounded state. Grab a notebook and a supportive friend or family member. Here is some basic hospice information so that when you have your meeting you can be better prepared.

Are there criteria to be a hospice patient?

Oh, yes. Most hospice programs follow the criteria set by Medicare (because the Medicare hospice benefit is the main funder for hospice). These guidelines are very strict and very specific. This is generally how it works.

> A doctor must refer you to hospice. This can happen in many ways. In Jenny's case, her oncologist recommended hospice after all her treatment options were exhausted. An emergency department physician may recommend hospice after your ninth visit to the ER with no response to your usual medical therapies. Or you or your family can initiate this conversation with your primary doctor if you feel like you are not doing well and the quality of your life has significantly diminished. This referring doctor will need to believe, in their best medical judgment, that you likely have six months or less to live if you let your disease run its natural course.

> You must meet criteria for hospice. The criteria are specific to your disease process or diagnosis and generally defined by Medicare regulations. For example, if you have end-stage liver disease, the doctor will look at your health history, specific labs (albumin, prothrombin time, INR, BUN, creatinine), your weight, and your appetite. They will also do a physical assessment to evaluate your overall health and determine how much care you need in a day. They will ask you about your goals for care and what is important to you. If you meet criteria based on the guidelines, they will refer you to hospice.

> A second physician must agree that you meet hospice criteria. The hospice doctor to whom you have been referred will also review your medical records and

possibly send a nurse to your home to assess you and evaluate your goals for care to determine if are eligible. The second doctor must agree in their best medical judgment, that you will die in the next six months if you let your disease run its natural course.

Finally, and most importantly, you must agree to hospice. You are ready to shift your medical care from cure to comfort. This means your medical providers will focus on managing your pain and symptoms and the quality of your life (*whatever that means to you*) rather than treating, curing, or fighting your disease. Hospice understands that this is a process and sometimes it takes patients a while and many conversations to make the decision.

What is hospice?

Hospice, in its best form, is the physical, spiritual, and emotional care of a human being at the end of one's life. Hospice care is still comprehensive and sophisticated medical care, but the focus becomes your comfort and the quality of your life—whatever that means to you. Your energy can shift from fighting your disease to formulating how you want to spend your last days, weeks, or months of your life. You and your family are the focus of hospice care.

Who is on the hospice team?

Your team consists of a physician, chaplain or spiritual counselor, social worker, nurse, home health aide, volunteer, and bereavement coordinator. You may not need all of these team members and you can certainly refuse any services (except for the nurse). Your team will meet about every two weeks to discuss and coordinate your care based on your personal goals.

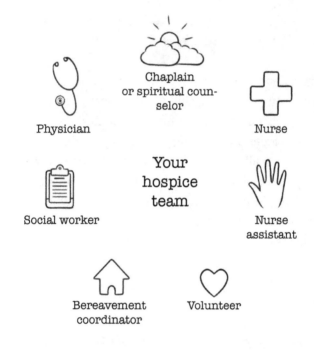

Physician

Chaplain or spiritual counselor

Nurse

Social worker

Your hospice team

Nurse assistant

Bereavement coordinator

Volunteer

Where does hospice happen?

Hospice is not a place, but rather a system of care that augments your personal caregivers. Your hospice team can visit you wherever you live. I have visited patients in the hospital, in their homes, nursing homes, foster homes, assisted living facilities, retirement homes, in an RV, and on a very tiny boat.

Most patients have hospice support in the comfort of their own home with family and friends as their primary caregiver(s). If you think your care cannot be managed at home, a social worker or case manager may be able to provide support as you and your family find other medically and financially realistic options such as private caregivers, nursing homes, or foster care homes.

Some hospice homes or facilities do exist. However, they may have very strict guidelines for financial reimbursement. You may not qualify to to stay there which is great news, it means your symptoms can be taken care of while you're still at home. I would definitely inquire if one is in your area.

When is hospice involved?

Hospice does not provide 24-hour care in the home. Hospice offers home visits on both a scheduled basis and when needed. You may have a nurse schedule visits two to three times a week and each visit may last about an hour, and you may choose to schedule a home health aide to assist you with your shower two times a week, or you may want the chaplain and/or social worker to meet with you weekly.

Hospice offers 24/7 advice and assistance by phone, and staff are available 24/7 for urgent needs. Issues arise all the time, so there's no need to feel apologetic about calling, even at 4 a.m. The night nurse has likely had four cups of coffee and is ready for a mission.

Who pays for hospice?

Generally, Medicare, Medicaid, and private insurances pay for hospice. Your potential hospice team can determine what your benefits will cover. If you don't have insurance, some hospices have funds to support those who need it.

Clarify with your doctor

Okay, now you have some basic information to formulate some questions. You can make better decisions about your care if you really understand your diagnosis, the benefits and burdens of continuing treatments, and options available to you. Remember, bring a friend and a notebook to the meeting. Ask the doctor any questions you have about your diagnosis. Why are you eligible for hospice now? What has changed? Ask them what it might look like if you choose hospice. What might it look like if you don't choose hospice?

Bring up any specific needs you want addressed, whether they be physical, emotional, spiritual, or even financial. Financial concerns can have an enormous impact on the quality of your life. What does your hospice insurance benefit cover? Who will take care of you? Can you stay in your home? What will that look like? Will there be any limitations on treatment that you are currently receiving?

When you are on hospice, some medical therapies may not be available to you any longer even though they may improve your comfort. For example, you may want to have radiation or chemotherapy while on hospice because this will ultimately help with pain management, or you may want weekly blood transfusions to improve your energy level. Some hospices cannot cover these expensive treatments, but others can do so.

If I choose hospice, is it still okay to have hope?

Yes! There is always hope. Hospice patients can stabilize. You may no longer meet criteria for hospice, in which case you will be discharged from hospice. I like to call this a graduation. My aunt has been on hospice four times and has graduated four times! I have witnessed many patients defy their medical prognoses, say goodbye to hospice, and live much longer than expected. You can also hope to be comfortable and to live a good life, even at the end of your life.

Can I change my mind about hospice?

You can choose to sign off of hospice at any time, and it will likely be available if you need it later. There is fine print involved in exiting and returning depending on your hospice benefit, but your hospice nurse or social worker can help you navigate it.

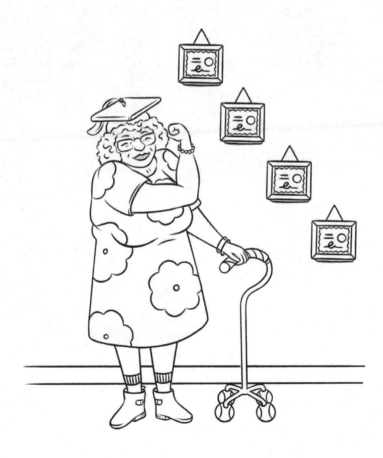

Arriving
in Mindful Presence

Coming into stillness

Take some moments to scan through your body

And just see what wants to relax, to let go a little

You might take a full deep in-breath

Filling the chest, filling the lungs

And a slow out-breath feeling the sensations of the breath as you release.

And again a deep in-breath

And a slow out-breath

Letting your breath then resume in its natural rhythm

Opening to your senses, feeling the breath in the foreground and relaxing with the background of sensations, sounds, feelings, and life.

Inspired by Tara Brach

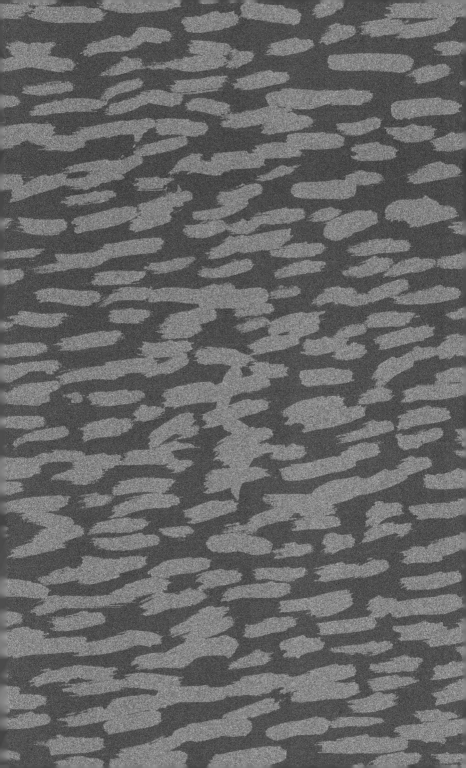

Opting

Out

Chapter 2:

Opting Out

When a doctor says you are ready for hospice—it doesn't mean *you* are ready for hospice. Many patients are focused on fighting their illness; they do not want to switch gears to "comfort care" and enthusiastically sign up with hospice. You may not be ready to stop the medical care you've become familiar with: treatment aimed at curing your disease, diagnostic tests, trips to the emergency room when your symptoms are unmanageable, and more hospitalizations. Many patients decline hospice. It's your choice.

If your doctor recommended hospice, it could mean that something has shifted in your disease process and perhaps you need to think differently about your care. I have seen many patients refuse hospice, increase their caregiving support and do much better.

If you opt out of hospice, consider the following.

> If you received a hospice referral, you may want to at least meet with the hospice so you can gather information and be in their system should your needs change or should you change your mind.
>
> Ask your medical provider if you have any other options beyond hospice to assist with your care.

Do you meet criteria for home health nursing visits? Generally, a patient needs to have acute nursing needs.

You may need to bolster your caregiving situation by asking family to check in more frequently or to live with you. You may need help getting dressed or with meal prep. This help can come as relief to anyone struggling with illness.

Perhaps you need a different living situation. Over the years I have met some ferociously independent patients who would literally crawl to the bathroom rather than ask for help. Maybe you need to live somewhere that has assistive care or 24/7 care, serves meals, and helps with dressing, bathing, bathroom trips, and laundry. Can your provider help you find the right care facility for you?

Ask your medical professional if home-based palliative care or an office-based palliative care program is available for you.

What is palliative care?

Palliative care is medical care provided to a patient with a serious or chronic illness such as lung disease, kidney failure, dementia, HIV, heart disease, or cancer. Life with a chronic illness can be overwhelming—your palliative care team can walk with you on this journey. Their availability and financial reimbursement may vary depending on where you are, your insurance or your specific disease. But in theory, from the moment you receive your diagnosis, they can provide emotional and spiritual support, resources, education, and symptom management. They work with you, your family, and your other medical providers as you receive treatment for your disease. And if needed, they can help you to land softly with a hospice team when your medical treatments are ineffective, or doing more harm than good, or you are significantly declining. You do not need a prognosis of six months or less to have a palliative care team, so patients may be able to access this medical team at any point in their illness. If available, a palliative care team is an excellent option.

I sometimes choose to ride my bike without a helmet. I make this choice because I love the feel of my hair blowing in the wind, I think I look cuter without a helmet, and I am literally going three miles an hour. Sometimes my neighbors yell, "Get your helmet on!" I want to yell back, "Let me make my own damn choices!" As you know, I am a fan of hospice, but I am also a fan of people making choices that are aligned with their own beliefs and values and spirit. Maybe hospice is not right for you right now, or maybe it will never be something you say yes to. That is okay. Our beautiful life is made up of our own damn choices.

Imagine how you want your surroundings to feel during the remainder of your life.

Discuss with a trusted person.

Choosing
Hospice

Chapter 3:
Choosing Hospice

There may be a point when you will be tired of fighting your disease, or you may not have any more medical therapies available to cure your illness, or you are declining and ready to switch to comfort care rather than curative or life-prolonging care. Choosing a hospice can be incredibly beneficial to patients and families at this time. Your hospice team will help you navigate your illness, manage any symptoms, and support you and your family. The goals are to maximize your comfort and the quality of your life at the end of your life. This chapter addresses how to choose a hospice and what your hospice team can offer. Bottom line: you want a hospice team that will answer the phone when you call, efficiently address your questions and concerns, expertly manage your symptoms, and work together to take care of you and your family.

You do have the right to choose any hospice agency, even if you have been referred to a specific hospice. Ask the physician why they referred you to this specific hospice and how it may benefit you. Their response may be satisfying and enough. Depending on where you live, you may or may not have a lot of hospice choices. If you do have many choices, it helps to do a little investigating.

Questions to consider when researching a hospice[1]

How is this hospice perceived in the community?
Though not always accurate, online research is one place to begin. Get references both from people you know and from people in the medical field, like hospital staff, nursing homes staff, or clinicians. Ask friends and family if they have had a recent experience. The quality of a hospice can sway significantly depending on leadership, financial resources available, and staff turnover. Did your friend have a good experience? How was their hospice helpful?

Are their doctors and nurses certified or credentialed in palliative care?
This reveals that they have studied and are knowledgeable in end-of-life care and symptom management.

Is the hospice Medicare-certified or accredited?
If Medicare is your primary insurance coverage, certification is essential for reimbursement. Accreditation shows that a third party has evaluated the hospice and it meets certain standards of care.

What does my hospice insurance benefit pay for?
Insurance coverage is legitimately confusing, so always ask if you have a hospice benefit and what your benefit will cover. Will your hospice benefit cover any extra therapies if they help with symptom relief such as palliative radiation or blood transfusions?

Any time your care needs change, whether you go to a hospital, a care center, an ER, or make any other changes, continue to ask about your insurance coverage.

How quickly can they respond to calls and requests for a home visit?

What is their triage system like during the day? How quickly will your nurse respond to your calls? If there is an emergency at 2 a.m. on a Sunday, who would they send and how long would it take?

What if your care is complex?

Some patients may require complex symptom management or have care needs beyond the scope of your family's abilities. Ask the hospice if they are equipped to handle your specific medical needs and how they would plan to address them. You will be surprised at how sophisticated hospice care is. If your symptoms become unmanageable in the home, the hospice should have a contract with a facility, hospital, or nursing home that will provide short term 24/7 nursing care to alleviate symptoms and manage care. When your symptoms are alleviated, you may be discharged back to your home. This is called general inpatient care. It may be helpful to know where the facility is located and if this stay is covered by your hospice benefit.

Hospice also may offer "continuous care" in your home for a limited time when you are in crisis. It is an option that can help you stay in your home while your symptoms are expertly managed. But again, it's important to know continuous care is for a limited time.

What is their plan for respite care?

When caregivers need a break, hospices offer "respite" care which can last up to five days. The patient would be moved to a facility, a nursing home, or foster home while the caregiver takes care of themselves. Ask the hospice where this care would take place.

How will they handle your concerns about the hospice?

If you have frustrations with your team, you will want to let the agency know. Is there a system in place to address any concerns? Ask about their process for handling problems.

How do they treat their staff?

When employees are valued and treated with respect and dignity, that care transfers to you.

What kind of bereavement services does the hospice offer?

Types of caregiver grief support after you have died can vary widely and may include individual counseling, support groups, educational materials, and outreach letters.

What is your overall impression?

You're going to share an intimate part of your life and your journey with this care team. Ideally they will be people you feel good about having around during this time. It's okay to trust your gut.

[1] Adapted with permission from www.americanhospice.org

Do I really need a hospice team?

The word "team" may sound a little daunting, but when a person is dying, it can be helpful to have professionals skilled in specific areas who can address your physical issues, your spiritual concerns, and your emotional needs. You can use this section as a guide when evaluating your potential team of caregivers and to advocate for yourself if your team isn't working for you. Let's take some time to get to know how these roles might function in their ideal form.

Hospice Doctor (MD/DO)
When you are on hospice, a physician will oversee your medical care. You may choose your personal physician or the hospice doctor to do this. Hospice doctors are specialists in managing end-of-life symptoms, understanding your personal medical needs, and supporting you as a whole person. Technically, a hospice doctor may or may not be "boarded" in hospice and palliative medicine. Boarded means they have specifically studied and taken exams in hospice and palliative care. Many hospice doctors are boarded in their prior area of focus, such as family medicine.

Personal Doctor (MD/DO)
It is possible to keep your current primary care physician or another doctor you are close to, such as your oncologist or cardiologist, involved in your care. Just ask them or your hospice team how to do this.

Nurse (RN)
Hospice nurses are experts at end-of-life care, managing your symptoms, and they will be your first responders for any medical

questions or concerns. You can tell them what is important to you and they can advocate for you. Each nurse has a trunk filled with gloves, catheters, supplies, a stethoscope, and, if they're smart, water and some protein bars.

Social Worker (MSW)
Social Workers can help you navigate anything that may concern you at the end of life: emotions, fears, family conflicts, caregiving, finances, living situation, grief, kids, community resources, aftercare planning, and bereavement needs. They are beyond resourceful. You can turn to them at any time.

Home Health Aide/Nurse Assistant
Home Health Aides help you with personal hygiene, grooming, light housekeeping, and overall care. They can bathe a bedbound patient while miraculously changing linens and braiding the patient's hair all at the same time. Sometimes these professionals are just the magic you need.

Interfaith Chaplain/Spiritual Counselor
Chaplains can help you connect to your religion or spirituality or provide counseling when you have existential questions that often arise near the end of life. While chaplains are generally rooted in a particular religious tradition, they are educated in serving people of all different cultural and faith backgrounds. Even if you don't define yourself as religious or spiritual, you could benefit from their emotional support. Chaplains can also educate your hospice team about your beliefs and traditions and offer bedside rituals that align with your beliefs—or they will find someone who can.

Volunteer

Weekly volunteers can broaden your support network. They can visit with you, play games, chat, sing, listen, and help out as needed. Many hospices offer specialty volunteers as well for music, art, massage, aromatherapy, and pet care.

Bereavement

Your caregivers may want to consider grief counseling and support after you have died. Hospices generally offer these services free for up to one year.

Each staff member should consider your needs holistically. If you are in pain when the home health aide gives you a bed bath, the aide should contact the nurse and let them know your pain is not well managed. If the nurse is taking your blood pressure and you mention you want last rites from your church, the nurse can make that happen. If the chaplain is praying with you and you mention your partner is mentally exhausted, they can initiate a conversation about respite care so your caregiver can have a break. If your expectations don't meet with the reality of your care, these descriptions can be a baseline for you to self-advocate.

Preparing
Your Affairs

You may want to spend some time preparing your affairs as it will eliminate confusion and free your family from the burden of making decisions for you. Or you may want to spend this time enjoying each moment with your family or enjoying the sun on your face. Some people do not get the chance to "prepare their affairs" and honestly, it's okay if you don't. Many people have died without their affairs in order.

If you wish to prepare, here is a list of a few things to consider sooner than later while you are in a physical and mental position to address them. You may need some help from your hospice team, medical professionals, family, or friends.

Appoint someone to be your decision-maker, health care representative, or official power of attorney (POA). This person can make decisions for you when you are unable to communicate.

If your state has this available, ask your doctor to complete a Physician Orders for Life-Sustaining

Treatment (POLST) to clarify your wishes for life support in an emergency situation.

Finish your will. (Or start it, as the case may be.)

Have frank and thoughtful discussions with your executor about your will. Transparency may help preserve relationships down the road. Remember: the executor will be the one to deal with all family members and any unforeseen injustices or unrealistic distribution of goods.

If it's important to you, consider sharing how you will want your family to handle your physical belongings.

Gather together your passwords for important accounts. Make a list of your online accounts to either have a trusted representative deactivate, unsubscribe, or delete the accounts.

Pick a funeral home. Online reviews can help, but be sure to ask around. You may want one near your home as your family may need to visit the funeral home.

Discuss your wishes for your funeral arrangements. You can plan for favorite songs, anointing, or spiritual rituals.

Consider how you want your loved ones to remember you. Share these wishes with your friends and family.

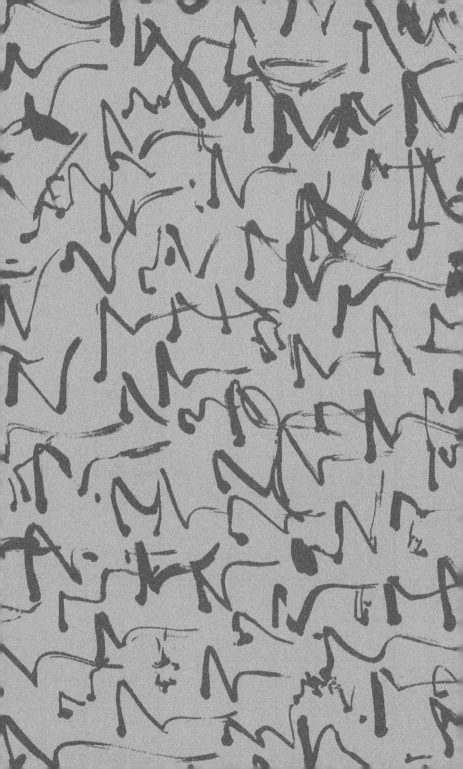

Consider one thing you wish to do before you die.

Enlist someone to help you complete your wish.

Choices

Chapter 4:
Choices

As a nurse, I feel it is important that I share some end-of-life options that may be available to you so you can make fully informed decisions about your care. It is also important that I respect your choices knowing they reflect your culture, religious beliefs, financial situation, family circumstances, and personal values. Here are some options you may want to be aware of so you can seek more information if needed to make thoughtful choices about your care.

Advance directive

You can fill out an "advance directive" form that will explicitly state your wishes if you are in a life-threatening circumstance and you cannot communicate. Each state has its own form, but in general you can make decisions about life support options (CPR, ventilators, and artificial nutrition or "tube feeding"). You can choose to have all medical interventions available to prevent or delay your death for as long as possible or you may want no intervention at all to allow death to come naturally or you can choose something in between.

Filling out an advance directive is an incredible gift to give to your family and friends, because then they don't have to guess at what you would want to do. I have supported many families during a crisis, and it is distressing to make these choices about tube feeding and ventilators for someone you love. If you make the decisions ahead of time, they can honor your wishes—whatever they are.

Appoint a health care agent
You can appoint a health care agent (usually simultaneously while filling out an advance directive form). Circumstances change all the time during a medical crisis and situations may arise that you could never anticipate. This person will make health care decisions if you are unable to do so, based on your values, beliefs, and what "quality of life" means to you.

Right to refuse or stop any medical therapy
As you have the right to initiate a therapy that your doctor offers which may provide some medical benefit, you also have the right to refuse or stop any medical therapy that may prolong your life or that you don't want. Life-prolonging medical therapies might include oxygen, dialysis, pacemakers, surgery, cancer treatments, ventilator support, antibiotics, tube-feeding, or artificial hydration (IV fluids). You will want to talk to your medical provider about this as medical and emotional support will be critical.

For instance, I've had patients request to be taken off oxygen when they are dying. When we do this, we have medications to alleviate shortness of breath (opioids), and we slowly turn down the oxygen while watching for any breathing difficulties. The goal is comfort at all times. So, if needed, we increase the medications over time (to ensure comfort) as the oxygen is slowly turned down. The patient will then remain on that medication to prevent labored breathing until they die.

Voluntarily stopping eating and drinking
Some patients with a terminal illness choose to not eat or drink anything as a way to speed up their death. If you are considering

this, please discuss your plan with your hospice team or medical provider so you have the proper information to make this decision. Your team can offer both medical support to minimize any discomfort and emotional support for you and your family.

It will require discipline and you will likely need someone to stay with you 24/7 if you choose this path, due to your anticipated weakness. It's always hard to predict when someone will die, and depending on your circumstances, you may survive days or weeks.

Medical aid in dying

Medical aid in dying (also known as "death with dignity" or "physician aid in dying") is legal in some states and jurisdictions. This statute allows qualified terminally ill adults to receive a prescription for life-ending medication they can take to bring about their imminent death. The patient criteria and regulations are strict and vary state by state. It takes an average of three to six weeks until someone can receive the prescription, and your out-of-pocket expense will vary depending on your insurance and medical coverage. Many patients do have hospice support simultaneously as they pursue this option. If it is legal in your state and you are considering medical aid in dying, ask your hospice provider if they support patients who want to research this end-of-life option as some do not.

When someone is diagnosed with a life-threatening illness, the rules, beliefs, and values that once governed their life may change. If you want more information about your health care choices, talk to your medical provider or hospice team. You can also request family conferences with these skilled professionals in the room to educate and inform all parties, as your family may have differing values and opinions regarding your care. Ultimately, these decisions are yours to make.

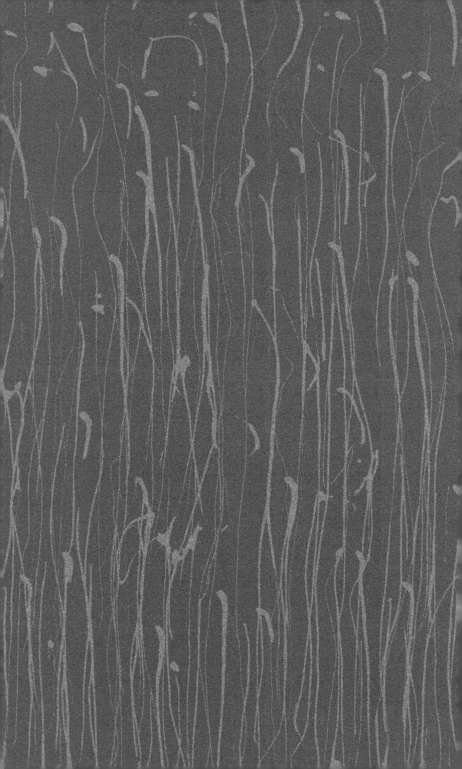

Make a list

of people

you trust.

Your

Care

Chapter 5:
Your Care

By now, you have either chosen a hospice team or you have a medical provider you can call for any medical concerns. It's time to think about who your personal caregivers will be. It takes all kinds of people to care for terminally ill patients, and I have seen the gamut: partners, parents, nieces, grown children, young children, friends, exes, coworkers, and siblings. When my mom revealed she was ready to sign up with hospice, our family looked at each other like, "You do it."

Mom essentially had six of us clueless caregivers, each with differing opinions. I was a freshly minted nurse, newly pregnant. My sisters and brothers all worked. And my dad's primary motivation was to "get mom off the morphine and get her better." We were a family that happy-houred together. We didn't exactly work together.

Thankfully, we had hospice support. They guided us and answered our calls. Mom connected with the social worker, probably as a result of discussing her negligent crew of family caregivers. We cooked and cleaned and made her milkshakes. We sat at her bedside as we planned my sister's wedding. Looking back, I am deeply grateful for the time we had with her: the laughs, the tears, even the fatigue. We didn't give my mom exquisite care, but we did give her loving care.

Assemble your team

Because your hospice team does not live with you, you will need help. If not yet, eventually. At minimum, have one go-to person. More often than not, your caregiving team is your family, and because family can be very, well, family, you may want to cast a wider net. Now is the time to cash in your favors and call your friends.

What if your living situation isn't ideal?

You may not have caregivers available, or you may require care beyond the scope of your family and friends' abilities. Ask your medical provider to refer you to someone who can help. A social worker may provide you and your family with information and resources, as you find medically and financially realistic options for your care such as private paid caregivers, nursing homes, or foster homes.

Discuss your needs

When constructing your team, consider your family culture. At this stage of your illness, you likely already know who is reliable and who is, ahem, less so. Have a frank discussion with anyone who will be giving you care.

Tell them the truth about your medical condition, your prognosis, and your needs. Ask them for honesty in return. Point out who is carrying the weight, and let the rest know how they can contribute. You can say something like this: "I am dying. I need help from everyone. I know you are all very busy but I need someone to be available for me on Mondays and Saturdays. Your sister, the one taking a nap on the ground next to the fridge, is exhausted because she has taken on a lot of my care and she's a little fried. It's time for everyone to step up." If you need to, ask for someone you trust to help you navigate this family-wide conversation.

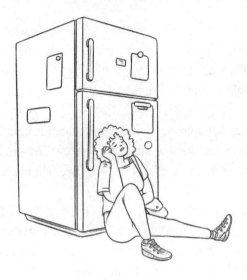

Assign roles

Some helpers will love having a job to do. They will feel empowered having a tangible action plan. Try assigning these roles:

> On-call 24/7 Contact
> Shopper
> Appointment Tracker
> Medication Manager
> Meal Planner
> Driver
> Grocery Getter
> Medical Contact

You can also assign each care person a day (or two or three) when they will help you or check in with you. Ideally, your team should be making your life easier and more comfortable.

Try tech support

If you have it, use technology to help organize your care.

Create a group text of two to seven people whom you can call upon when needed: "I need some almond milk, a pill crusher, and a nice bottle of cabernet." Might as well ask, right?

Use a spreadsheet to make a medication chart, with the name, dosages, and times taken. Low-tech version: keep track of medications in a notebook.

Use video chat services like Skype or FaceTime to connect with people. It may help you preserve your energy or stay connected to people across the world for whom a visit may be impossible.

Try using a central calendar for all of your appointments and visits. Hospice will likely schedule days and times so you can use a calendar to manage your full care plan. Low-tech version: make a central handwritten or printed calendar to put on the fridge.

Program medication times and alerts into your phone if you have trouble remembering to take them on time. It may be helpful to organize your pills into small containers for the week.

Start meal delivery

Ask friends and family to start a meal delivery for you. It will do more than just alleviate the need to cook. It's a low-impact way to maintain a connection with others. People want to help and to feel needed. If you belong to a faith organization, ask them to chip in.

Meal drop-off does not necessarily mean drop anchor. Let these lovely volunteers know you may not have the energy to chat when they bring the casserole. If you aren't up for visitors, place a cooler outside the door for drop-off. Request disposable dishes or establish a pick-up system. If you do not have anyone you can ask, your hospice social worker or medical provider may be able to connect you with meal programs that exist in your area.

What do I need?

Consider the following items and send your selected shopper on their mission:

> A notebook is critical. You will want to keep track of medication times and when they were given, bowel movements, and perhaps phone conversations. You will forget. If you have different caregivers, such tracking helps everyone get on the same page.

> Latex gloves. If you need them, you'll be glad to have them on hand.

> A soft blanket.

> Tissues. Get the fluffy ones.

> Games, art and drawing supplies, puzzles, or other "quiet time" activities that don't require screen time. Use these to connect with people when you don't want to talk about death or dying. (That topic gets old fast, and it's uncomfortable for some.)

> Chocolate. Or whatever you like to treat yourself with.

> A bell to rouse tired caregivers.

> Comfortable, soft, stretchy pajamas.
>
> Streaming video service. Movies can be an enjoyable distraction when you are weary.
>
> Streaming music. Use music to shift the energy in the room. Some days, this journey can feel sad, so perhaps some jazz would elevate your spirits, or maybe today you want to steep in your mood.

Let your caregivers help so you can conserve your energy for enjoyable tasks. Your personal team cares about you and wants you to be your happiest and most comfortable. Don't be afraid to manage them, and ask for what you need to make yourself feel better. These are probably the last few months of your life. If you want the window open or some brie cheese, go ahead and ask.

Caregiver's Tip ─────────────────────

Be kind and gentle to the hospice patient.

Your loved one is losing control of their surroundings, their health, and life as they know it. Everything is shifting—their work identity, their role in their family or society, their ability to travel, their financial and physical independence. Perhaps they cannot eat foods they once loved, perhaps they cannot connect with people in the way they once did. They may be grappling with their own death and the mystery on the other side of this life. Dying is so personal and it may feel very isolating. And physically, they may be in pain or short of breath or nauseated. They may react differently than they have in the past.

Offer the patient control and choice whenever you can. Admire their grace. Be in awe when they smile at you. Offer reverence and lots of love. Slow down. Their life is moving much slower than yours. Sit next to them. Offer to hold their hand. Be okay with not talking. Hold their space with grace and tenderness, the best you can. If you need help or assistance, please ask for it.

Be kind and gentle with your caregivers.

Try to put yourself in your caregiver's well-worn shoes. It takes incredible strength and grace to take care of a family member or friend who is dying. Their entire universe is shifting painfully along with yours. They are taking care of you and managing everything else (laundry, food, finances, etc.). They are probably tired, lonely, and quietly grieving.

Based on my experiences of talking with caregivers after their loved ones have died, your caregiver will never regret taking care of you. However, to maintain their compassion and kind-heartedness, they may need to step out and do some yoga, lie down, cry, watch a movie, and take a day or two or ten off. When they are taking care of themselves, they can take better care of you.

I know it's hard to ask for help, but you will want and need assistance at the end of your life. When my mom asked me to take care of her, I was terrified. I look back on my life of 50 years and still say taking care of my mom was one of the greatest things I have ever done. It was clunky and awkward and tiring at times, but 100 percent without a doubt, the greatest gift my mom ever gave me.

Record a conversation about what has changed over your lifetime.

Discuss what you hope will change in the world.

Visitors

Chapter 6:

Visitors

Human connection can be essential at end of life for the terminal patient and the visitor. This chapter addresses how patients can maintain some control and not be overwhelmed by visits, and reminds the visitor to respect the patient's wishes.

Caregiver's Tip ───────────────────────────

Caregivers, family, and friends: be mindful of your own opinions, values, and religious beliefs when you visit a hospice patient.

Ask what is important to them, and respect their answer, whatever it is. Request permission to say prayers, to set up salt lamps, install a children's choir, or change their environment. The patient may say, "No thank you," and it's their choice.

One of my first-ever hospice patients was lying in bed watching soap operas all day long. I suggested to my nurse mentor that perhaps we could turn the TV off and play some soothing music. She said, "Beth, she loves soap operas and she gets to choose whatever she wants. This is her final chapter to write—not yours." Ouch. But a critical reminder to leave my own preferences at the door.

When should family and friends come to visit?

I usually advise for visits sooner rather than later because you just never know how long someone has. You are probably more able to engage in meaningful conversations and impart your pearls of wisdom now—so now is a better time than later.

Establish limits, if necessary. Consider what is your most energetic time of the day and try to schedule visits during this time. You can enlist a bouncer to enforce your rules, e.g., one visitor at a time for fifteen minutes each. Have a chair available and ask for your visitor to sit so they can relax and be eye-level with you.

If you're afraid of pain, anxiety, or nausea during the visit, you can try pre-medicating to ensure your symptoms are under control. If

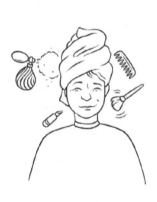

you're afraid of looking "too sick" or just not your best, enlist help to look like your radiant self. A home health aide can make you sparkle.

If you do agree to visitors, it can impact them for a long time, maybe for the rest of their lives. They will be so grateful they visited you whether it was three months, one month, or one day before you died. If you are having a rough day and you are not up for visitors, just say that.

What if a relative or friend cannot visit?

If your friends or family can't visit due to time constraints or finances, there are other ways to connect. Talk to your friends and family on the phone or video chat. They will appreciate the opportunity to articulate how much they love you and how much you mean to them. If you are too tired to speak, have someone hold the phone to your ear, or set up your computer, and let your relative do the talking.

What if I don't want to see anyone?

Of course, you don't have to see anyone, or a specific someone, and that's okay.

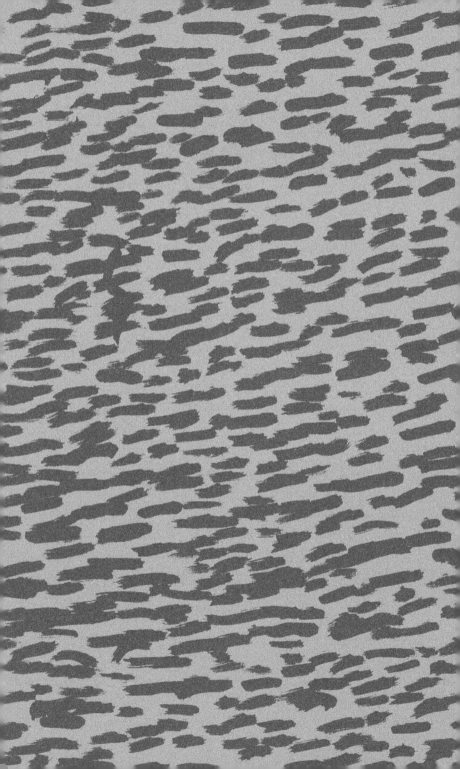

Abandon
a tradition
that no
    longer
serves you.

Energy & Mobility

Chapter 7:
Energy & Mobility

Stella was a vibrant 80-year-old—tiny and sassy—but her morning shower took the wind out of her sails. She slept the remainder of the day, unable to visit with anyone. Stella finally agreed to a bed bath, and we saw her quality of life markedly improve. She now had the energy to joke with the staff, watch her favorite cat videos, and visit with her family in the sun.

That's a much more satisfying day than sleeping.

As you decline, you will likely experience changes in your energy and mobility. This section should help you navigate the changes that may become a part of your daily experience.

Hospice nurses get these same questions all the time:

> Should I get a hospital bed? (Probably.)
>
> I want to go outside but cannot independently. Should I? (Yes, let's try.)
>
> Can my grandchild crawl into bed with me? (Hmm, this one depends on the kid.)

How can I stay energetic?

Your daily energy level will fluctuate, and that may be frustrating. Talk to your medical provider or hospice team. They may have ideas, medications, or equipment that can help to increase your energy.

Do what your body allows you to do, for as long as you can or want

This helps to maintain strength and independence. Move your body if it feels good and right. Bend limbs, stretch, rotate wrists and ankles. Walk. Enlist support. Try to get outside for some fresh air. Mobility will help with everything: mood, change of scenery, joints, muscle aches, circulation, and constipation.

Conserve your energy for events that make you the happiest

If your energy is waning, consider which tasks are boring or exhausting (e.g., showering, getting dressed, making breakfast, eating, etc.) and ask for help or delegate some tasks to your team during these times. Schedule fun events (visitors, outings, art) at your favorite and most energetic time of the day.

Try to stay on a regular sleep cycle

It's easier to have caregivers that are awake at the same time you are. That said, if you want to nap during the day, nap away. No one should ever call you lazy. It's okay to rest if you need it.

Consider using medical equipment

Sometimes, the best way to maintain your energy is to use medical equipment like a hospital bed, a wheelchair, or a bedside commode. Usually, your hospice insurance benefit covers certain medical equipment, and your hospice team can help you to obtain any items so you don't have to buy or rent them. You can try them out, and if they don't work for you, you can return them.

A hospital bed can be placed wherever you wish as long as you have the space. (Beds are approximately thirty-eight inches by eighty-four inches and may or may not include twin sheets.) The head of the bed can be raised up mechanically, which is useful for dining in bed and getting out of bed. The entire bed can be elevated straight up so your caregivers don't compromise their backs while trying to change the linens or bathe you. You will need your caregivers functioning at maximum capacity.

A wheelchair expands your universe. You may not realize that, over time, your life has shrunk to a twenty-foot radius due to weakness. You don't go outside anymore. You haven't seen the kitchen in days. A wheelchair may be what allows you to stroll around the neighborhood or go on a more adventurous outing with the family.

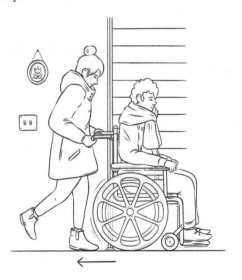

I recommend that your primary wheelchair driver play with the equipment first before you jump into the wheelchair. There are practical ways to navigate thresholds and curbs (big wheels first over bumps and down curbs). Consider the width of your hallways, as many homes are not wheelchair accessible.

A bedside commode provides ease-of-access when the toilet feels far, far away, and can be especially helpful if you're tethered to an oxygen system or other medical equipment. You can set up the commode near the bed, walk a few steps, and pee. Your caregiver can clean it out, squirt some deodorizer, and voilà: you're back to bed.

Set up a little handwashing station with a basin filled with warm, sudsy water and a dry washcloth. Consider purchasing absorbent pads for the bed when you become less mobile as accidents can happen.

Conserving your energy allows you to partake in the more enjoyable bits of life: watching an NBA game, crushing your granddaughter at Mario Kart, or drinking a nice glass of cabernet, shared with your best friend.

What if I'm too tired to get out of bed or become "bedbound"?

One day, you may try to get out of bed and simply cannot. It's frustrating when your body is no longer listening to your brain and your heart. If your fatigue wins today, don't despair. Energy levels often shift at this time and you may feel more energetic tomorrow. Most patients are so determined to get out of bed despite their weak bodies, but this can be unsafe, both for you and your caregiver.

If your loved one insists on getting out of bed but cannot safely do so.

You can say, "Mom, your body is just too tired to get up today. It's not safe for you and it's not safe for my back. Let's get back to bed and try again tomorrow."

As you spend more time in bed, you will definitely need more help. Ask your good people to be available 24/7. Just because you have to stay in bed doesn't mean you have to give up on your happiness. I recommend the following tasks to maximize your comfort and control.

Modify your environment

Pull a table nearer to your bed for ready access to things you want. If you're going to be in bed, make your space as perfect as it can be. Ask some- one to bring you eyeglasses, tissues, snacks, remote control, magazines, tiny bouquet of flowers, your tablet, cellphone, scotch, and maybe a bell to rouse your sleepy caregiver. Whatever will give you some peace and enjoyment.

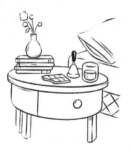

Ask your friends to sit

Always have a chair available for someone to sit next to you. It can be a strange—even hierarchical—dynamic to have people standing over you at your bedside. Having your visitors sit allows for eye engagement, and prevents you from craning your neck or staring at your friend's waist.

Tidy up
Better yet, ask others to tidy up for you.

I popped in to check on my mom one morning when she was bedbound. She growled, "Why doesn't anyone see that damn envelope sitting in the corner? It has been there for days." My mom never complained about anything. Sure enough, there was a damn envelope sitting in the corner that had likely been there for days, maybe weeks. The room feels smaller with each passing day, so ask your friends and family to tidy up when they leave.

Establish a routine
It can be very disorienting to be in bed all day. In the morning, open the curtains and the windows for a bit of light and fresh air. Ask someone to help you get ready for the day. Wash your face and hands. Brush your teeth. If you have hair, brush it every day. Set meal times may help to provide structure in your day.

Get comfortable
Now that your space and routine are feeling good, it's time to get comfy. Ask your team to help you.

> If you want, accept offers for back rubs or light massage. Keep lotion nearby, as this can keep your skin supple, and the massage stimulates circulation.

Practice gentle range of motion exercises or stretches, even while in bed, to keep your joints agile and prevent stiffness. Lift your arms, bend your legs, rotate your wrists and ankles, and so on.

Gather some extra pillows for positioning and maximum comfort. Ask your caregivers to help eliminate any wrinkles in your sheets or clothing; even a small one can feel mind-numbingly annoying.

Find soft, stretchy clothing. If you're having trouble dressing, cut the back side of your shirt or gown three-quarters of the way up (along the line of your backbone). This way you can get dressed in one simple motion and eliminate the uncomfortable wrinkle issue.

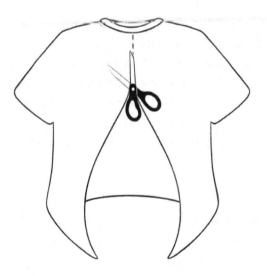

Plan ahead for the need to urinate and have bowel movements while in bed

Staying in bed can be difficult physically but really takes a mental toll. This is where the rubber meets the road. For urgency's sake, let's get practical first and process later. You will want absorbent pads under you at this time. It will alleviate the need for a full linen change if you have an accident in bed. Your caregiver will need wipes, latex gloves, a basin, soap, and washcloths.

You may want to use a bedpan/urinal

Ask your hospice team if they have these items and can bring them to you and offer instructions on how to best use. The bedpan is for women to urinate or have a bowel movement. Men can use a urinal to urinate and a bedpan to have a bowel movement.

Consider using "briefs"

I prefer the more distinguished term "briefs" for "adult diapers." No one likes the idea of urinating in a brief, but it may even be more comfortable than sitting on a bedpan if you can believe it. Check your briefs every four hours or so while awake to ensure you are clean and dry. There is a lot of rolling involved when you are changed in bed and you will need a caregiver or two to do this for you.

Inquire about a catheter

This is a tube inserted into your urethra to drain your urine. A catheter can help eliminate the overall discomfort and moisture that urine can present. It also minimizes the number of brief-changing episodes (which can be exhausting) and allows you to conserve your energy for more enjoyable tasks.

Each option is annoying in its own way, and may feel like it's chipping away at your integrity, so make the choice that provides you with the most comfort and dignity.

You may want to talk to someone you trust about this loss of control and independence. These are major issues at this stage of an illness. Your hospice team may be able to compassionately support you and listen to the struggle. Because this struggle is as real as it gets.

Can kids and pets get into bed with me?

That's up to you. You are in control. If you are having pain or if your grandchild is the ninja-warrior type, I don't recommend it. Younger people may not have the right amount of sensitivity around touch and play for your body, especially if you are experiencing pain.

Can I sleep with a partner if I'm bedbound?

Everyone should consent first, of course, and then yes. You can and should sleep with whomever you wish. You may need help moving over to one side of the bed—hospital beds are built for singles—but then let the sparks begin—or not. It's up to you. Just snoozing together can be a very sweet connection.

How can I prevent bedsores?

When lying in bed for too long, certain body parts may be susceptible to pressure injuries, also known as "bedsores." Even a tiny one hurts like hell. Here are some prevention tips that may help. Common injury sites are the tailbone, elbows, back of the head, heels, ears, and hips, if you lie on your side.

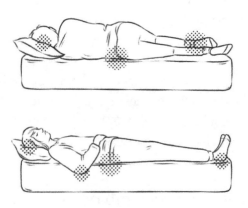

Regularly inspect these susceptible spots. If the site has a reddish hue and you touch it and it doesn't turn white ("non-blanching"), be a little more vigilant about repositioning your body so that you have less pressure on this red area.

Regularly inspect and protect the skin in contact with medical devices and lines

Pressure injuries can also occur from nasal cannulas, tracheostomy ties, breathing masks, or other devices. If you experience discomfort in these areas or see redness, talk to your hospice team or medical provider for suggestions to prevent skin breakdown.

Reposition

Reposition yourself or have your caregiver reposition you every two to four hours or so while you're awake, using pillows to relieve pressure. Ask your team for guidance on how to safely reposition.

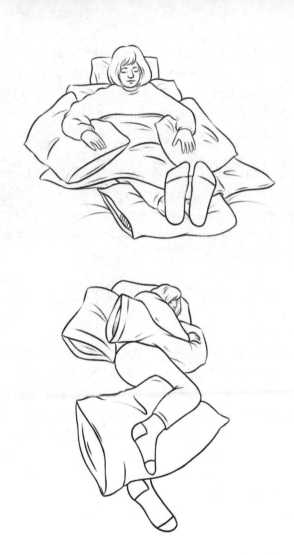

Ask someone to apply lotion

Have your caregiver try warming up lotion in a basin of warm water prior to use and gently massage some into your skin. This helps increase circulation and can elevate your skin to a radiant glow.

If you're hungry, eat protein-rich and fatty foods
These foods facilitate wound healing, but what you eat is up to you. Your wishes are the most important. Though I have seen spectacular results with wounds healing at the end of life, major wound healing at this time is not generally expected.

Unfortunately, even if you and/or your caregiver strictly adhere to these suggestions, you may get a bedsore no matter what. If this happens, I absolve you and your caregiver from any guilt they may experience. The skin is an organ and may simply break down at this stage.

How can I stay clean and dry?

Ask for bed baths
Baths are serious business and should not be taken lightly. When a patient is in bed all day and used to taking showers they will feel like a camper—dirty and sad (which is why I don't camp). Consider asking the home health aide to give you a bed bath and change your linens two to three times a week. Additionally, you will need new linens if they become moist from sweat or other fluids. Bathing someone in a bed is actually an acquired skill. Here is one method.

Caregiver's Tip _____

You will want several towels, a basin with warm water, a cup for rinsing, a warm blanket or two, a few wet washcloths, a few dry washcloths, possibly no rinse shampoo or soap. Start at the head. Place a large towel gently under the head. Slowly, wet hair with a small cup of warm water, shielding eyes, and gently scrub shampoo into head. Get the back of the head. Rinse as you go.

Gently dry with washcloth or small towel. Comb their hair. Place a dry towel under the patient's head. Now move from the face down the body only cleaning their front side. Gently wash and dry as you go and make sure the patient is warm enough along the way. Scrub those armpits and apply deodorant. Clean and dry their private areas gently but thoroughly (using different washcloths and water for this area). Continue on to the toes.

Apply a warm blanket to their front. Have the patient roll to one side. Wash and dry from top to toes again using separate washcloths and water for the bottom zone. Roll to the other side and repeat. Add fresh clothes and underwear, and you are good to go.

What if I'm desperate to move?

So, your room is tidy and your bed is comfy, but you still feel stuck. Looking at the same four walls—same everything—can get old, fast. Ask your caregivers if they can change the bed's position or location. Can they move it slightly so it's easier to see out the window? And while they are at it, can someone put a bird feeder outside your window? Sometimes simply changing your view can be a huge improvement on the quality of your day.

What if I want to go outside?

Most hospital beds have wheels, so, if you have a large door frame or double doors, it's possible to move the bed outside. In my experience, it is never easy, and generally, door frames get slightly mangled, but it is almost always worth it.

You can also be carried to the outdoors, but you must assess the cost-benefit analysis. Is it worth the risk?

I regret that we didn't move my mom from her bedroom with the damn envelope once she was bedbound. My mom was tiny, probably all of 80 pounds. I'm five feet one, but I carried my 80-pound kids around when they were flailing and crying for God's sake. My mom would have been quiet and still and grateful. I can only imagine how it might have improved her mood or completely shifted the tone of her day if I'd carried her outdoors. So, if all parties feel up for it, give it a try.

Over time you will get weaker and more fatigued. You will eventually stay in bed more and sleep more. This is frustrating for most patients and you may need to process this with someone. You can still have a robust personality and have fun even as your energy wanes. You can still boss everyone around or be filled with gratitude, or both. You can still have thoughtful conversations, be angry at politicians, enjoy your granddaughter's drawing, or be moved to tears by a passage from a holy book. Though your world is getting physically smaller, your life can still be big and meaningful, whatever that means to you.

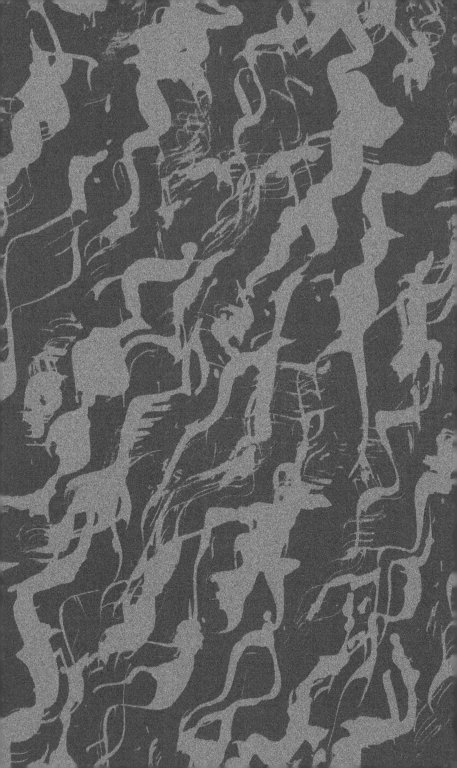

Allow

yourself

to laugh.

Eating

& Drinking

Chapter 8:
Eating & Drinking

Your relationship with food and beverages will look very different during different stages of your illness. This section will help you navigate the changes as you decline over time. In general, I recommend eating and drinking whatever the hell you want while you are still able, because eating is fun and will raise your energy level and your spirit. Even if you have always lived with dietary restrictions, now may be the time to say yes to milkshakes, yes to chocolate, and yes to tequila.

In general, you should maintain control of what you eat and drink because you are the only one who truly knows if you are hungry or thirsty, and you'll be in touch with how your digestive system is working. If you do not want to eat, you can say, "No thank you." If you're craving an ice cream sundae in the morning, do it. Many cultures express love through food, so it can be very hard for some family and friends to accept that you are not hungry or do not crave your typical foods. Your team can offer you food and beverages throughout the day and help if you need assistance, but no one should pressure you to eat or drink. If you are frustrated that your appetite is waning, sometimes certain medications can help to increase your appetite, so talk to your hospice team or medical provider.

Satisfying, easy to eat foods

Though I am a fan of eating whatever the hell you want, certain foods can help you feel better, heal wounds, and stabilize your energy level throughout the day.

Have foods that are prepped, satisfying, and easy to eat, like freshly sliced watermelon, bananas, peaches, applesauce, popsicles, full fat yogurt, ice cream, soups, avocado slices. Consider easy-to-eat proteins like lentils, fish, tofu, roasted chicken, or eggs. Any type of potato—yams, russets, purple potatoes—cooked or mashed are rich and satisfying. Add butter to increase caloric intake (and joy). Fermented foods like kefir or miso can aid in digestion. Whole grains like oatmeal, brown rice, and cooked vegetables (roasted or sautéed in olive oil) can pack in some nutrition while generally being easy to swallow. Nutritional drinks or shakes may also assist you in boosting your caloric and protein intake.

When should I eat?

Whenever you want.

If mealtime is important to you, establish routines. It may help to add structure to your day, and it may give friends or family the opportunity to feel like life is somewhat normal. You may not want to eat what they're eating, but you can partake in the conversation and ritual. Alternatively, you can eat small, frequent meals throughout the day. I call this "grazing."

As time goes on, you may experience a decreased appetite. That's because you have different nutritional requirements now. For instance, if you're spending more time in bed, you're expending fewer calories than your caregiver (who has probably completed ten thousand steps by 8 a.m.). A decreased appetite is the body's natural way of eliminating unnecessary work. So don't be surprised if you decide you actually don't want to eat that burger in front of you.

What if it's hard to swallow?

Food may become difficult to swallow. Your head and heart may want to eat pizza, but your body may not. Food intake may require a cost/benefit analysis. Does the benefit of enjoyment outweigh the discomfort afterwards? Only you can know for sure.

If you cough and sputter with each attempt to eat, consider foods that easily slide down the throat like those recommended: popsicles, slippery fresh fruit, applesauce, yogurt, soups, ice cream, milkshakes, or Jell-O. When eating, sit upright, at ninety degrees or so. Tuck your chin when you swallow. If those foods are difficult to swallow try ice chips, bits of popsicles, using a spoon, or liquids through an oral syringe.

If you are still coughing or choking, stop for a bit. Maybe it's not safe for you to eat or drink today. You can try again later. Diminished intake is a natural part of this process.

Oral care is still very important at this time. Keep your teeth, mouth, and gums clean and moist. Use an oral syringe, or a mouth swab to moisten/clean your mouth. Apply lip balm.

IV Fluids

Intravenous (IV) fluids are fluids that are administered through a small tube into your vein allowing a person to be artificially hydrated, among other things. Generally, IV fluids are not recommended for those on hospice. Decreased appetite and decreased thirst are a normal part of the dying process and a natural way for the body to eliminate unnecessary work. Your organs are retiring. Excess fluids in your body could potentially be more harmful than beneficial when your kidneys are slowing down, which may lead to uncomfortable symptoms such as swelling in your legs or shortness of breath. If you have questions, ask your hospice team or provider.

Over time your appetite will wane, your body will have fewer caloric needs, and it may become physically difficult to swallow. These are all natural parts of the dying process, but can be emotionally difficult to get on board with. Keep your family apprised of what you need and what you want. I had one patient request meat loaf from a favorite restaurant in his last days and the smell of it was enough to make him happy. Another requested watermelon popsicles and another just wanted coffee on a mouth swab. Though small, these moments will continue to make up your sweet and savory life.

Continue a mealtime ritual

whether or not you are eating.

Managing Your

Medications

Chapter 9:

Managing Your Medications

Managing your medications, especially if you are not in the medical field, can be a hair-raising experience. If family is now taking care of your medications, it may be difficult to let go of the control and trust they actually know what they are doing. This chapter provides some basic information on tracking, administration, and medication safety.

Keeping track of your medications is crucial. Write down your medications, their purpose (pain, nausea, etc.), scheduled times, and when they were administered in a notebook or spreadsheet. That way, if you have multiple caregivers, they can easily see what has been given and when, and your hospice team can also easily review your medications. Your team may decide to increase your pain medication, or they may consider a long-acting pain management solution based on your records. (Sample chart in this chapter).

Try to establish a convenient medication regimen. Schedule critical meds, (e.g., for pain control, shortness of breath, nausea, anxiety, and agitation) at times that work for you, like 9 a.m. and 9 p.m. or perhaps noon and midnight. Wake up to take these critical meds. Make it easy to take your medications by organizing your pills in medication containers for the week. If you are overwhelmed by the number of medications you have to swallow in a day, consider eliminating the ones that may not support you at this time such as vitamin D, fish oil, cholesterol pills, etc. You must talk to your hospice team or medical professional before making these decisions.

How long will it take for my medications to be effective?

When you are experiencing a distressing symptom such as nausea, pain, or anxiety, many patients want to know how long you have to wait until a medication starts working. How and where ("route") you administer your medications will determine when the medication reaches its optimal effectiveness ("peak") and how long it will last ("expected duration"). You will feel the effects of your medication before the "peak" time, but you should expect to see the best results from your medication at the peak time noted in the chart in this chapter. It's important to wait until the peak time to determine if it is an effective dose for you. Call your hospice team or medical provider if your symptom is not managed at the peak time, or if the medication does not last the entire expected duration.

Medication	Route	Peak	Duration
Pill or tablet	Oral	1 hour	3-4 hours
Pill/long-acting medication (e.g., MS Contin & Oxycontin)	Oral	4 hours	8-12 hours
Sublingual/under the tongue/slurry in the cheek: similar to oral pill	Oral	1 hour	3-4 hours
Rectal medication or suppository	Rectal	1 hour	3-4 hours

Patch (e.g., fentanyl patch)	Patch	24-72 hours after first patch is applied	Each patch should last 72 hours
IV Medication	IV	5-15 minutes	1-4 hours
Subcutaneous route	Like an IV but inserted under the skin	30 minutes	1-4 hours

Though there are definitely exceptions and variability depending on your body and the actual medication, in general you can expect something like this. Please double check with your team regarding specific medications.

Let's say your pain is awful, a 10/10 on the pain scale. You take your oral pain medication at 6 a.m. By 6:30 a.m., your pain will hopefully begin to subside. If at 7 a.m., peak time, your pain is still distressing to you at a 5/10 on the pain scale, call your hospice team or doctor.

If, however, at 7 a.m., your pain medication brings your pain down to a 2/10 on the pain scale, and that is acceptable to you, but does not last the entire four hours (expected duration), you should call your hospice team or medical provider.

Your team should continue to advise you, either in person or over the phone, until your pain is relieved.

Medication Safety
Always call your hospice team or medical provider with any medication concerns.

Never adjust medication doses on your own.
You may need a change in dosage or a different medication altogether if your medication...

is not managing your symptom.

is causing distressing side effects (nausea, over-whelming fatigue).

does not effectively relieve your symptom at the peak time or is not effective for the entire expected duration.

When your medical provider/hospice team prescribes a certain medication and specific dose, they consider many variables such as your illness, where your medication is metabolized (kidneys, lungs, gut, or liver), your age, or if you are "naïve" to this drug (have never had it before). If you do not follow what has been prescribed, there may be some pretty unappealing consequences.

You may suffer damage to your kidneys or liver.

Prescriptions may run out sooner than anticipated.

The medical provider or hospice team will not have accurate information to sufficiently or safely increase or decrease your dose.

Do not assume you can crush any pill.
Some pills should not be crushed. For example, if MS Contin (extended release morphine) is crushed, you will receive the entire dose in a very short time, and this is dangerous. Ask your hospice team, medical provider, or pharmacist before you crush a pill.

Sample Chart

Scheduled Medication	Reason	Instructions & dosage	Time scheduled	Date/Time taken & Notes						
				M 7/20	T 7/21	W 7/22	T 7/23	F 7/24	S 7/25	S 7/26
Fentanyl patch	Pain	apply 50 mcg patch every 72 hours to rotating areas on skin	9 am, every 72 hours	9 am (applied to right chest)			8:30 am (applied to left upper arm)			9:30 am (applied to left chest)
Senokot	Prevent constipation	1 tablet every morning	9 am	8 am	9 am	10 am	9:15 am	8:30 am	9 am	9 am

As-needed Medication	Reason	Instructions & dosage	Frequency							
				M 7/20	T 7/21	W 7/22	T 7/23	F 7/24	S 7/25	S 7/26
Morphine liquid intensol	Pain	take 5 mg (25 mls) as needed for pain, place in mouth or inside cheek	Every 1 hour as needed	7 am 5 mg	3 am 5 mg, 7 am 5 mg, 8 am 5 mg, 2 pm 5 mg	noon 5 mg	9 pm 5 mg	noon 5 mg 1 pm 5 mg	9 am 5 mg	
Compazine	Nausea	10 mg as needed	Every 8 hours as needed				8 am	9 am		
Tylenol	Pain, fever	take 2 325 mg tabs (650 mg total) every 6 hours as needed	Every 6 hours as needed	6 pm (2 tabs)	10 pm (2 tabs)		noon (2 tabs) 6 pm (2 tabs)			

When should I premedicate?

Try to anticipate events that cause you pain, anxiety, nausea, or shortness of breath. Schedule your medication times to coincide when the drug will be most effective. For instance, if you always have pain when you shower, take a dose of pain medicine one hour before you shower. If you experience shortness of breath when you go outside for your morning walk, take your oral medication that helps with shortness of breath one hour before you walk.

What are some ways to take medications when it's difficult to swallow?

Try a whole pill in a "slippery" food: applesauce, ice cream, pudding, or yogurt. If that doesn't work, crush the pill and mix with a slippery food. (Remember: some pills should not be crushed.)

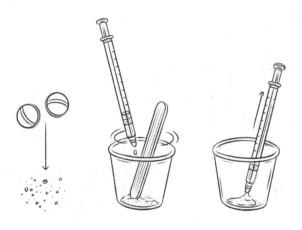

If neither of these options works, try a "slurry." Crush your pill and place crushed contents in a medication cup. Place beverage of choice (water, apple juice, soda) in another cup. Draw up a tiny amount of beverage in an oral syringe and mix that fluid with the crushed contents of the pill. Gently and slowly insert this mixture into your mouth between your cheek and gums. Consider adding honey, cherry syrup, or chocolate syrup to further mask the bitterness.

If you cannot safely swallow, call your hospice team or medical provider. They may change your medicine to a liquid form or they may instruct you or your caregiver on how to give your medication rectally. When my mom couldn't swallow and had to take her MS Contin rectally, I asked, "Um, and who perchance will administer this drug?" (Remember, I am a nurse). Hospice was very nonchalant about it: "Oh, you will, honey." Well, I did it and it was fine—I was just a little bit grumpy that no one appreciated the significance of the job and my mom's lovely attitude about it.

Caregiver's Tip _____

How to insert a medication rectally

1. Get permission from the patient.
2. Wash and dry your hands.
3. If medication is wrapped, unwrap it!
4. Put on gloves.
5. If available, place some water-soluble lubricant on the tip of the suppository or the pill.
6. Ask patient to lie on their side (left side if you are administering an enema).
7. Spread the butt cheeks and slide the suppository/medication gently into the rectum about one inch.
8. Remove your gloves.

9. Cover patient back up.

Optional: Apologize for their discomfort.

Not Optional: Wash your hands.

Most patients and families are apprehensive about taking on the role of nurse and pharmacist in the home, but you do have backup—your hospice team or medical provider—to call with questions or concerns. And honestly, you will be amazed at what your family and friends can do! If you feel your medical care and symptoms cannot be effectively managed in the home, call to ask about other options available at this time.

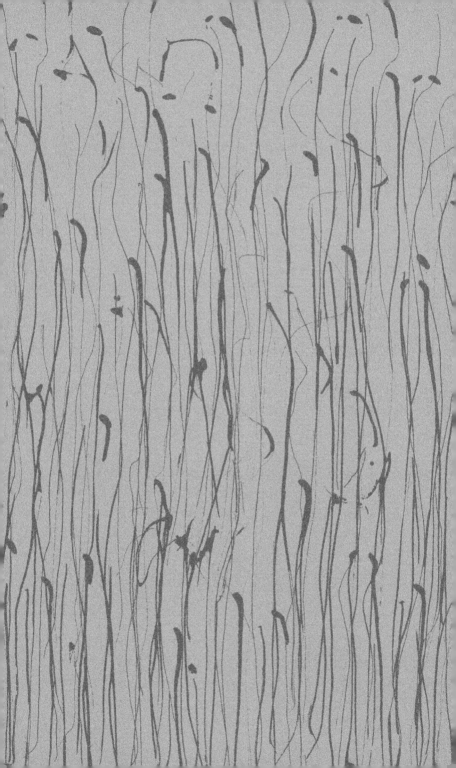

Identify a project or task you want someone

to carry on after you no longer can.

Pain

Chapter 10:
Pain

S tanding by when a patient is miserable may be the most challenging part of being a caregiver. You are bearing witness to their suffering. You will need to show up with all of your love and an understanding that you cannot take away their suffering. It is a tough balancing act.

Pull up a chair next to the bed and sit down. Offer gentle reassurance. If you are waiting for medications to kick in, keep an eye on the time to help assess if the medications are working as expected. If they are not working, call the hospice team. Practice being present. Relax your body. And breathe. Showing up, being present—this is love.

Try a breathing exercise

Tune in to your toes. Get grounded. Feel your body.

Inhale. 1, 2, 3, 4.

Relax any tension as you...

Exhale. 1, 2, 3, 4.

If your mind wanders or you want to flee, gently bring yourself back to the present. This helps to build up your compassion muscles. Continue to breathe in this manner.

At end of life, you may or may not develop certain aggravating physical symptoms. I addressed some common issues that may occur. I think it helps to have some basic information and an understanding as to why your hospice team prescribes certain drugs. When you are not in the medical field, all of the medications can sound exactly the same. "Take this oxymorphicodyl...blah blah blah." And if you haven't slept and are nauseated or in pain, nothing makes much sense in the moment. Your hospice team or medical provider is especially skilled at managing your symptoms—and contact with them will be critical to your ongoing support and education.

—

Anyone who has had significant pain knows that it can affect you physically, yes, but also socially, spiritually, and emotionally. When your pain is well controlled, everything in your life looks a lot better and brighter. One key goal of hospice is to prevent and decrease pain in the easiest way possible.

When I asked one gentleman about his pain, he tensely replied, "I'm fine if I don't move."

"Well," I said, "what is important to you? Do you want to stay in bed today?"

"My granddaughter is coming in a bit," he replied, "and, at some point, I will probably have to use the bathroom."

"You have pain medicine prescribed to you," I reminded him. "You can start with the smallest dose and you should start feeling better within an hour."

He hesitated, but agreed to try it. After about half an hour, the smile came back to his face. After an hour, he was visibly relaxed and able to get out of bed to visit with his granddaughter when she arrived.

How will hospice manage my pain?

Hospice practitioners are experts at pain management. Medications are chosen for you depending on many variables: your illness, age, medical history, kidney and liver function, and practical considerations, such as cost, where you live, and who is administering the drug.

Your medical provider may initially prescribe a non-opioid such as acetaminophen (Tylenol) or ibuprofen (Advil or Motrin).

If non-opioids alone are not enough to manage your pain, your hospice team or medical provider may prescribe an opioid. Opioids are a type of narcotic. They include prescription medicine like oxycodone and morphine and you will need ongoing medical guidance.

Adjuvants are excellent additions to one's pain regimen because they do not have the same side effects of opioids, and they may help to limit the use of opioids overall. They may be prescribed in addition to your typical pain regimen. Adjuvant pain medications can include antidepressants, anti-seizure medications, muscle relaxants, sedatives, or anti-anxiety medications. Their primary function is generally not used for pain management but is effective in alleviating certain types of pain (e.g., bone pain or nerve pain) and/or the fear and anxiety that may accompany pain.

If your pain increases or varies wildly throughout the day, your medical provider may then prescribe a long-acting opioid or schedule pain medications around the clock to allow for more consistent relief. The goal is to prevent pain.

Opioids commonly prescribed for pain include:

MSIR: morphine sulfate immediate release tablets

Roxanol: highly concentrated liquid morphine

MS Contin: long-acting morphine

Oxycodone: short-acting oxycodone

Oxycontin: long-acting oxycodone

Lortab/Norco: hydrocodone + acetaminophen

Methadone: used as a short-acting or long-acting pain reliever

Dilaudid: hydromorphone

Duragesic: fentanyl patch

How do I verbally describe my pain?

Your hospice team will consistently ask you about your pain. Tell your team when it hurts, where it hurts, and how bad your pain is. Descriptive words can help your medical team determine which type of medication you need. For example, if you say it's "burning pain," you may need a medication for nerve pain.

It can be hard for patients to articulate their pain in words. Many pain scales exist, but the ones I've found to be most effective in eliciting a response are the 0–10 scale, Mild Pain vs. Moderate vs. Severe Pain scales, or the simple question, "Can you tell me about your pain?"

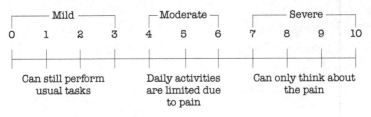

Mild — 0 1 2 3 | Moderate — 4 5 6 | Severe — 7 8 9 10

Can still perform usual tasks | Daily activities are limited due to pain | Can only think about the pain

Caregiver's Tip

Always believe the patient when they say they are in pain. No matter what.

What if I don't want to or cannot describe my pain?

If you don't want to or cannot describe your pain, families and caregivers should look for these indicators:

> grimacing (clenched teeth, expression of concern)

> frowning

furrowed brow (brows come together)

crying

moaning

groaning

grunting

labored breathing (fast, maybe deep breathing—it will look like you are struggling to breathe.)

tension in the body or face

clenched fist

knees pulled up

guarding parts of the body—for example, if your stomach hurts you will block (guard) your stomach with your arm to make sure no one touches this body part.

refusing to move

withdrawal—less responsive, not talking with others as you normally would

irritability

agitation

When should I take pain medication?

Take your pain medication when it's scheduled to be taken. If your hospice team or medical provider has prescribed you pain medication to take **as needed ("PRN")**, take it when...

> Your pain is a three or four on the 0–10 pain scale. Don't wait until it's a 10 out of 10.
>
> Pain is mild, but you are thinking about it.
>
> You have something to do in an hour, but you are afraid to do it because of pain.

How can I anticipate my pain?

If you have pain with certain types of activity like showering, walking, or turning, you should premedicate. For instance, if you often have pain in the shower, take your prescribed dose of oral pain medication one hour before you shower.

Is there any reason I should *not* take pain medications?

As a hospice nurse, I always recommend pain medications over suffering, but many people have firm beliefs against taking medication. I often tell my patients that this pain (cancer pain, nerve pain, bone pain) is different than any other type of pain—because it probably is. This kind of pain requires a different approach than a normal headache. You can always start with the smallest dose and see how you respond to it. Most people are surprised by how much better their life is when they have their pain controlled.

What are the side effects of opioids?

Typical side effects of opioids include constipation, sleepiness, nausea, rash, itching, hallucinations, and slower breathing. With the exception of constipation, these side effects should improve within a few days to weeks of starting the opioid. If your opioid is causing troubling side effects, call your hospice team or medical provider. One opioid may make you nauseated but another may not. It may be helpful to try a different opioid if recommended by your team. Please call your team to discuss any of these side effects.

Why do I need a laxative when I take opioids?

When you take opioids, they slow down the natural movement of the intestine. You will definitely get constipated and it won't go away unless you take laxatives.

You should take the laxatives before you become constipated for them to be effective. Don't wait until you haven't pooped in a week. (See Ch. 11.)

What if I feel sleepy when on pain medications?

Patients and families are often bothered by the sleepiness that may be caused by pain medications. Not everyone gets sleepy when they take an opioid, and sometimes patients may actually have more energy because their pain is finally well-managed. It usually takes a few days for the opioid to reach a stable level in your body and then you should become more alert again. It's important to let your family and team know how you feel about your alertness. Some patients may welcome the sleep over the pain they have been experiencing, or they may want to be alert every moment of the day no matter how awful their pain is.

A critical question for you: Would you rather be alert and in pain or sleepy with less pain? Your answer to this question may change daily. Consider this question often and communicate your preferences with your family and caregivers.

Should I fear getting addicted to an opioid?

Hospice patients who are in pain take opioids because they need them. In hospice, we start with the lowest dose and increase medications slowly and safely, if needed. You may develop a tolerance over time. This doesn't mean you are addicted. It means that your previous dose is not effective any more. If you have concerns, please talk to your hospice team, medical provider, or a counselor if you have one.

What about substance abuse?

Hospice can work with people who are currently struggling with or have a history of substance abuse. Sometimes, people in recovery are worried about taking opioids at the end of their life. Your hospice doctor is an expert in pain management—they know how to handle this. If current substance abuse is suspected, your hospice will typically provide a medication contract to which you must abide, a lock box for medications, and lots of emotional support. Consider discussing any concerns with a hospice team member.

Can my emotions worsen my pain?

Yes, they can. Consider the emotions that may accompany your pain: anxiety, anger, fear, loneliness, or boredom. Being with others who care about you may be the most critical solution at this time—ask a friend, family member, or someone from your hospice team to sit with you and discuss your concerns.

How can I manage my pain without medication?

Distractions
Watch TV, make art, cuddle with furry pet friends, listen to music, change your scenery, watch cat videos.

Presence
Have a friend sit next to you. If you wish, consider eliminating cell phones or laptops from your room at this time.

Therapeutic touch
Gentle massage. Apply warm lotion.

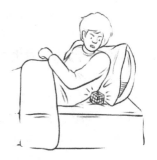

Change your position
You may find the source of the pain.

Reading
Have someone read your favorite passage, book, or a poem that soothes you.

Going outside
Breathe some fresh air.

Other methods
If available, use acupuncture, reiki, or craniosacral therapy. These complementary therapies may help with many other symptoms too—such as anxiety, fear, and nausea.

Marijuana

Medical marijuana is legal in many states and may require a recommendation from a medical doctor or doctor of osteopathy, and/or a medical card to obtain it. Patients sometimes use marijuana for symptoms such as pain, nausea, appetite, and anxiety. Ask your hospice team if they can recommend any resources for you.

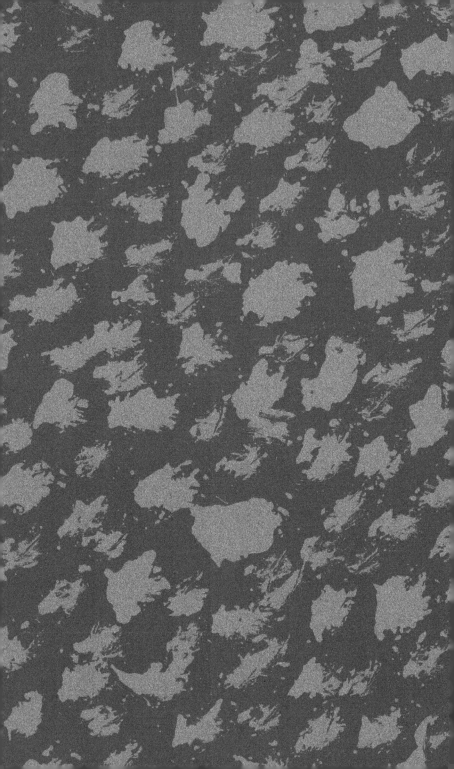

Read
out loud.

Constipation

Chapter 11:

Constipation

Hospice nurses are obsessed with bowel movements, also known as pooping. Constipation is when you have too few bowel movements in a week, you experience difficulty when you have a bowel movement, or you simply cannot have a bowel movement. It's important to keep your bowels moving and prevent constipation as it can lead to pain or nausea and vomiting.

You have approximately twenty feet of small bowel and five feet of colon—the lining of your colon is constantly regenerating, which is why you still need to have bowel movements. You should have a bowel movement at least every three days, even if you aren't eating or drinking much or anything at all. Your hospice nurse will ask you about your bowel movements at each visit, so you may want to document the day you had a bowel movement and the size of your bowel movement. Otherwise, you may forget.

The causes of constipation are many. Generally, if you are on hospice, using opioids may be the primary cause. Opioids stop the gut from working—end of story. If you're on an opioid, you will need to be on laxatives (sometimes two or three) starting as soon as you start your opioid.

Some common pharmaceutical interventions prescribed to prevent constipation are:

Senokot: senna

MiraLAX: polyethylene glycol

Enulose: lactulose

Dulcolax: bisacodyl

Fleet enema: sodium phosphates

Colace: docusate sodium

How can I help prevent constipation?

Increase your fluid intake.

Increase your movement. Consider taking a walk.

Practice gentle abdominal massage.

Drink warm prune juice.

If you are not drinking enough fluids and are using fiber supplements, the fiber product may do more harm than good. Think cement.

Take your medications as prescribed.

If laxatives are not working or you have not had a bowel movement in three days or you experience nausea, vomiting, bloating, or poor appetite, call your hospice team or medical provider.

Change
the mood
of the room
with music.

Anxiety

Chapter 12:

Anxiety

Anxiety is common. Most hospices will provide medicines for anxiety when a patient signs on to hospice. Consider what is causing your anxiety because various causes of anxiety have different solutions.

Are you anxious because you have a scheduled visit from your (adorable) ninja warrior grandkids? Ask them to come over later, or on another day. Time your antianxiety medication promptly at 3 p.m., so, when they arrive at 4 p.m., you will care less when they start drawing with a Sharpie on the dining room table. You can gift them said dining room table in your will.

Are you anxious because you're afraid that your pain is getting out of control? Stay on top of your pain medications. Take pain medication when you are at a three or four on the 10-point pain scale.

Are you anxious because you're fearful of death? Talk to someone about your fears. Have a conversation with the chaplain, nurse, social worker, a family member, or take time to pray or meditate. Many of our questions about death don't have any logical answers, and we simply have to sit in the murky mystery of it all. We all need some support and help to process these big questions.

What medications can help my anxiety?

Everyone is different and your unique biochemistry may do well with a certain type of antianxiety medication, or it may not.

Keep talking with your hospice team and medical provider about what is working and what is not. They may recommend one of these commonly used anti-anxiety medications:

> Ativan: lorazepam

> Valium: diazepam

How can I control my anxiety without using medications?

Create a low-stimulation environment: a quiet room, dim lights, hushed tones. Consider whether you want to have a cell phone and laptop-free zone. Thumping on a keyboard or scrolling on screens may increase your agitation. I would want to turn the news off, but I have seen many patients who feel a sense of calm when it's on. It's all about setting up a soothing environment.

> Allow only one or two visitors at a time, and consider setting a time limit on each visit. Anxiety breeds anxiety. You may not be anxious, but Auntie Em just had four cups of coffee and is nervously pacing around your bedroom. You can kindly ask her to leave.
>
> If you are able, go for a walk. This may alleviate nervous energy.
>
> Put on some music that calms you.

Ask for a foot massage.

Wrap up in a warm blanket right out of the dryer. Or if you're hot, step outside for some air.

Meditate or pray.

Focus on your breath, the inhale and the exhale. Repeat.

Establish a centering ritual for stressful times. Light a candle, or listen to a restful song. Find a mantra, a phrase, or a word that helps to center or calm you.

Body Scan

This is written assuming you are in a chair. Please alter the meditation if you are lying down. Try asking someone to read it aloud to you the first few times you try it. Eventually you may be able to recall the steps on your own.

Begin by bringing your attention into your body.

You can close your eyes if that's comfortable for you.

You can notice your body seated wherever you're seated, feeling the weight of your body on the chair, on the floor.

Take a few deep breaths.

You can notice your feet on the floor, notice the sensations of your feet touching the floor. The weight and pressure, vibration, heat, and other obvious sensations.

You can notice your legs against the chair, pressure, pulsing, heaviness, lightness.

Notice your back against the chair.

Bring your attention into your stomach area. If your stomach is tense or tight, let it soften. Take a breath. We often hold a lot of tension in our stomach area.

Notice your hands. Can you feel vibrations, tingling, lightness, or heaviness? Are your hands tense or tight? See if you can allow them to soften.

Notice your arms. Feel any sensation in your arms. Let your shoulders be soft.

Notice your neck and throat. Let them be soft. Relax.

Soften your jaw. Let your face and facial muscles be soft.

Then notice your whole body present. Take one more breath.

Be aware of your whole body as best you can. Take a breath. And then when you're ready, you can open your eyes or end the meditation.

Produced by Diana Winston, Director of Mindfulness Education, UCLA's Mindful Awareness Research Center (MARC).

Shortness

of Breath

Chapter 13:
Shortness of Breath

I once visited a hospice patient who was living independently. After knocking several times, the social worker and I entered the open and unlocked door. She was sitting breathless, staring vacantly, and motioning us to her. We made her eggs and brought her water. She took a few bites and she slowly began to revive. She was so short of breath she couldn't get out of her chair to prepare food for herself or even close the front door. Shortness of breath is a debilitating symptom. When you can't breathe, it's difficult to talk, eat, and move. Life during this time can be exhausting—period. This exhaustion may lead to weight loss, decreased mobility, bedsores, the inability to socialize, and extreme boredom.

What if shortness of breath limits my mobility?

You may have already eliminated activities that cause shortness of breath, or you may be attached to an oxygen tank and only able to walk to your bed, bathroom, and perhaps a chair.

Here are some things you can do to make your life easier.

Conserve your energy (breathing) for tasks that are most enjoyable.

Modify your physical space by placing all necessary items within reach.

Arrange for meals that are prepared, easy to access, and require minimal chewing. Chewing can be surprisingly exhausting. (See food suggestions, Chapter 8.)

Be gentle with yourself. When you can't breathe well, it's normal to feel angry and panicky.

A wheelchair will help conserve your energy and may allow you to venture beyond your bedroom. You may need a driver for the wheelchair, if it takes too much energy to maneuver.

You may have oxygen tanks, concentrators, and tubing running throughout the house, or just in your room. Enlist help to make your room(s) safe for you and to remove tripping hazards to help prevent falls.

Never allow smoke or fire (including candles or cigarettes) when oxygen is in use. Use flameless candles for mood lighting or spiritual and ritual activities.

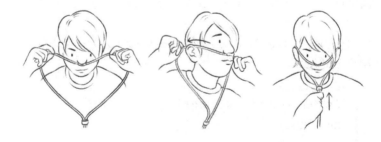

What can I do when I feel short of breath?

Turn on a fan. A fan blowing directly on your face helps diminish the feeling of "air hunger." This can be a game-changer.

Change your position. Sit upright in bed or in a chair. Or you may want to lean over a table. This helps your lungs expand.

Have pillows at your side, again, for greater lung expansion.

Keep the doors open. Many patients feel claustrophobic when short of breath.

If there is a nice breeze, open a window.

Move the bed toward the window to broaden your horizon.

If you are able, head outdoors for some fresh air.

If you're on oxygen, call your doctor to ask about turning up your oxygen. Certain diseases may get worse with an increase in oxygen, so please call first!

Breathe in through your nose and exhale slowly through your slightly closed lips.

Place a moist washcloth to your forehead.

Create a calm environment.

Consider turning off the news (unless no news adds to your panic).

What medications can help me with shortness of breath?

Call your hospice team or medical provider to determine if you have any medication you can take to alleviate shortness of breath.

Opioids
Opioids such as morphine are commonly prescribed to manage shortness of breath. Take the prescribed dose, and then wait. If you take your morphine at 2 a.m., you should be breathing easier by 3 a.m. (subtracting the fact that it's 3 a.m.). Your provider can start with the smallest dose to see if you tolerate it well and if it is effective for you.

Nebulizers/Inhalers.
Take as prescribed.

Antianxiety medications
When you are having trouble breathing, you may feel anxious as well. It's a vicious cycle: you can't breathe, so you get anxious, so you can't breathe, so you get anxious. If prescribed, antianxiety medications may help.

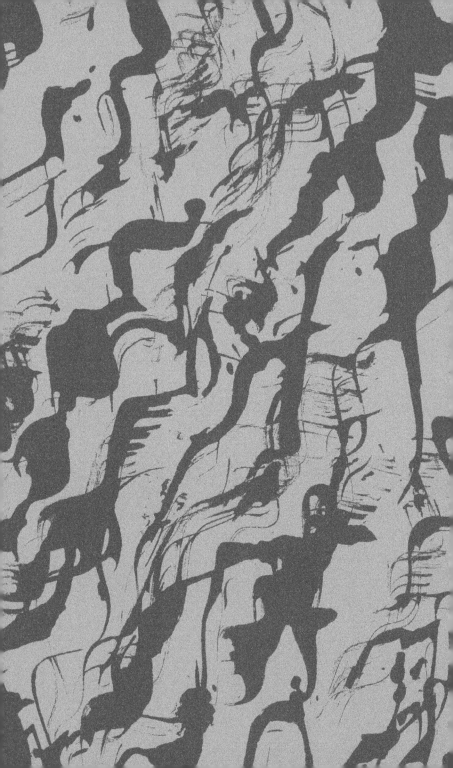

Write a letter
to your loved one.
Tell them when
you want them
to open it.

Nausea

& Vomiting

Chapter 14:

Nausea & Vomiting

There are many reasons why people have nausea or vomiting, and your doctor will prescribe specific medications for you based on why you are vomiting. Let your team know what is causing your nausea. For instance, anxiety, odors, medications, constipation, or movement/motion can all trigger nausea, and each cause requires a specific medication.

What medications can help me with nausea?

Common medicines prescribed for this include:

Haldol: haloperidol

Ativan: lorazepam

Compazine: prochlorperazine

Zofran: ondansetron

Reglan: metoclopramide

Benadryl: diphenhydramine

The same rules apply to routes of administration and peak effectiveness (noted in the section on medication management, chapter 9). So, a rectal anti-nausea medication may start working within 15 minutes and will peak in about an hour.

If you're having persistent nausea or vomiting, take the anti-nausea medication around the clock (per your medical provider's orders) until at least 24 to 48 hours after the nausea and vomiting stop. Talk with your hospice team or medical provider about this.

If you are vomiting, you probably cannot keep your pills down. Talk to your provider about another way to take your anti-nausea medication: rectal medications, the slurry method (see chapter 9), or, if available, subcutaneous injections (under the skin) or IV (into the vein) medications.

What else can I do to relieve my nausea/ vomiting?

Have you had a bowel movement in the last three days? If not, constipation could be causing your nausea or vomiting. Call your hospice or medical provider. You may need a suppository or enema.

Drink clear liquids for 24 hours to let your gut rest: broth, popsicles, apple juice, black coffee, and water.

Peppermint and ginger can help with nausea. Try taking them as a tea.

If you must eat, try bland, boring foods: bananas, rice, apple slices, toast. Yawn.

Keep your room cool.

Eat cool/cold foods.

Eat smaller portions.

Sit upright to help with swallowing.

Minimize odors. Tell your grandkids to cut back on the body spray.

Can I still eat food even if I vomit afterward?

Um, sure, if you want to. We call this "recreational eating." It just has to be worth it to you. Does the benefit outweigh the cost?

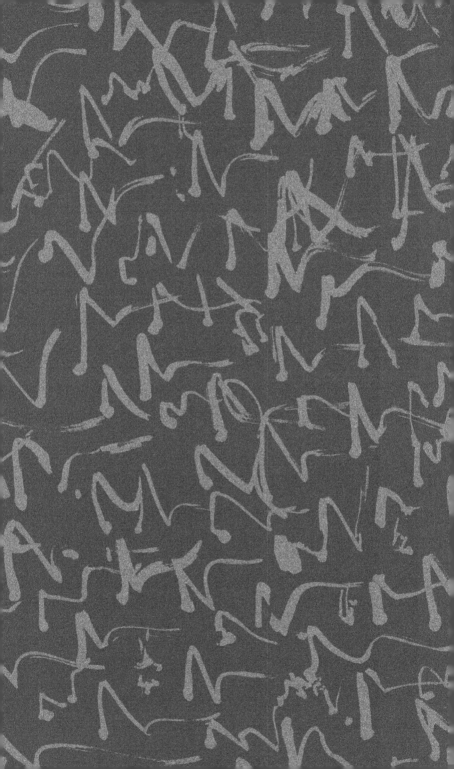

Tell a story

about something

you got away

with.

Confusion

& Delirium

Chapter 15:
Confusion & Delirium

Delirium is a state of sudden and often severe confusion that presents in many different ways. You may be unable to focus, your mind may be foggy, or you may alternate from sleepy to agitated and then return to your normal mental status. You may ramble, speak incoherently, or hallucinate. Delirium comes and goes. It is difficult to experience and to care for. If you think you are experiencing delirium, call your hospice team or medical provider sooner than later. Probably now. Caregivers should pay attention to the signs, as you may not be able to call for the help you need.

What do I need to consider if I have delirium?

You won't be thinking clearly all of the time and you will need help. You are not safe to be alone, and you will need someone to make decisions for you.

Caregiver's Tip _____

Consider Safety
Look at the room environment. What can be changed to prevent tripping or safety hazards? Consider 24/7 care as the patient is not thinking clearly. Sitting with the patient and gently reassuring

or reorienting may help.

Common reasons for delirium include constipation, extremely high or low blood sugar, infection, medications, trouble urinating, urinary catheters, low oxygen levels, pain, and decreased fluid intake. The good news is if the cause is discovered and treated effectively, your delirium may go away.

What medications help with delirium?

Haldol: haloperidol

Risperdal: risperidone

Zyprexa: olanzapine

Seroquel: quetiapine

Share what

you believe

happens when

someone dies.

Emergency

Room Visits

Chapter 16:

Emergency Room Visits

In a perfect world, hospice can manage most of your symptoms and circumstances at home, however a situation may arise and you want to go to the emergency room. If your instincts are to call 911 because something has happened at home—your pain is out of control, you are desperately short of breath—hospice generally prefers to be your first call during the emergency. Your hospice team or medical provider should be able to make recommendations over the phone and visit you. Most hospices have protocols in place for emergencies. If their recommendations do not work to resolve your crisis, they may suggest you go to an in-patient hospice facility or the emergency room. If your hospice team is not responsive or you can't wait, call 911 and reach out to your hospice team when you are able.

If an ER visit is recommended by the hospice team, the team will work to coordinate your ER visit prior to your arrival. If you have the documents, bring your POLST and Advance Directive to the ER; tell them you are a hospice patient and your goal is to be comfortable. The ER should have the tools to alleviate your symptoms without any extraordinary measures.

What are your goals?

When you are living with a terminal illness and facing an emergency your goals may get fuzzy. Some patients are very clear—they want minimal medical treatment—just keep them comfortable. To help clarify your goals, ask yourself, "What will I do with any new information I receive from x-rays, blood draws, and MRIs?" "Will my treatment change if they find my cancer has metastasized to another organ?" "Do I want to spend more time in the hospital?" "What is most important to me at this time?" Your hospice team or medical provider can help you understand the pros and cons of more treatment.

Example of emergency situations

I once cared for a gentleman with terminal cancer who suddenly developed symptoms of pneumonia. He decided he wanted to go to the hospital and receive IV antibiotics for the pneumonia to prolong his life, as the pneumonia may have caused him to die sooner. The patient stayed in the hospital for a few days then returned home with hospice support. Another hospice patient had kidney failure but suffered a broken hip from a fall. The patient and family decided not to surgically repair the bone, due to the high risk of surgery, and instead opted for increasing comfort care. He arrived at our in-patient facility to receive IV pain medications and was kept comfortable until he died.

What does my insurance cover?

If you decide to go to the emergency room, clarify what your hospice insurance benefit covers to prevent any financial surprises.

You may have to sign off hospice (hospice revocation) and resume your previous insurance benefit. Each situation is different, and payment depends on how your ER visit relates to your hospice diagnosis.

Can I resume hospice once my crisis has been managed in the ER or the hospital?

Yes. If you signed off of hospice (hospice revocation), you may have lost a hospice benefit period, but you should be able to sign back on to hospice when you are ready. It may be a good time to reconsider your goals of care. Is hospice still what you want? Do you want your care to be managed at home with hospice support? Or do you prefer to be hospitalized for symptoms or to use 911 as your emergency back-up rather than hospice. You can have a discussion with your family and/or your hospice team to clarify your wishes.

Tell a story about someone who has loved you.

Processing

Chapter 17:
Processing

To process your own mortality, especially when you are dying, is huge. Please take advantage of your hospice medical professionals, they are literally trained in this department. Ask them outright: Can you help me with my suffering? Can you help me find peace with my death? For some you may need to work through your anger at your cancer, for others you may wish to find inner forgiveness with a broken relationship, and others may want to make a video for their young daughter.

How do I emotionally process my terminal illness?

This time in your life is as raw and as real as it gets. Here are some suggestions for emotionally processing your death based on my experience watching from the sidelines.

Be gentle with yourself

Eat and sleep. My family can certainly vouch that I need these two items to be more emotionally, um, stable. Manage your pain. When your pain is controlled, you can access your higher state of well-being with greater ease.

Process
Talk to your hospice team, a priest, rabbi, chaplain, counselor, or friend—anyone you trust.

Pray or meditate
When life is feeling out of control, prayer or meditation can invite a sense of calm and hope and you can easily do it while lying down. You can pray to God, Allah, the great cosmos, Buddha, the creator, or your unconditionally loving dog. Find a soothing place. In your garden, in bed, in the bathtub, or wherever feels sacred to you. The simple act of asking for help can greatly shift one's mindset. When you are exhausted, you can ask someone else to read important passages to you or a guided meditation while you steep in the words and calm your nervous system.

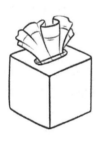

Cry
Tears are a significant part of this process.

If you aren't crying, someone else probably will be. So keep soft, fluffy tissues on hand—perhaps boxes of them.

Go ahead and lose your shit
It's okay to be angry. Anger is a normal part of processing something out of your control, so go ahead and let it out. I think it would feel very satisfying to break some plates if I had a terminal diagnosis—like, a lot of them.

Avoid

It might seem counterintuitive, but distractions can be great. When my mom was dying from lung cancer, she grew so tired of people bringing her books like Chicken Soup for the Cancer Soul. One day my husband and my mom perused design magazines and drank milkshakes while planning her future kitchen remodel. She appreciated the diversion and dreaming a bit.

Accept

Some days you will feel secure and pragmatic, saying, "Oh, yes, everyone dies...." This doesn't mean you're "giving up." Acceptance may give you relief, and if it reaches you, well, embrace it.

Feel it

When you acknowledge and feel your anxiety, fear, sadness, or anger, they may have less control over you and subside a bit. Guided meditation may help you in these moments.

Everyone processes their death differently. There is beauty in that. Trust that you'll do it in whatever way you need, and if you need help, call your hospice team or medical provider for suggestions or to request comforting and skilled support.

Caregiver's Tip

Listening is enough. It's perfect, in fact. Just sit down and sink into it. Practice being present. You do not need any answers to your loved one's questions, nor do you have to respond optimistically. You can say things like, "I don't know. That's a tough question." Or, "I am sorry for your sadness." Or you can sit in supportive silence.

What should I say to my loved ones?

If you have always been quiet or stoic, no one expects you to suddenly become emotionally transparent and effusive about your relationships. However, a terminal illness does give you and your family and friends some time for closure while you are living. In *The Four Things That Matter Most*, Ira Byock offers simple phrases that may help mend and nurture relationships at any time, but especially at the end of life:

> "Please forgive me."
>
> "I forgive you."
>
> "Thank you."
>
> "I love you."

These simple but critical phrases can encourage deeper discussion and may help to maintain a sweet connection after you have died. These phrases can clear the path for all parties to eventually say goodbye. If these don't feel quite right, you might try to think about what phrasing is right for each relationship or what message is important to convey. What do you need to say?

I have witnessed family members who were estranged come together and just hug or cry or sit without any words exchanged.

I have also seen hard honesty delivered during this difficult time soften relationships.

Though I am a proponent of seeking to heal relationships at this time, you may not want to see a specific someone, and that is okay. Maybe you want to send a blessing their way. A simple gesture can sometimes bring about great healing for the sender. Or maybe not. Some relationships are beyond repair and it's okay to say, *I forgive you* to yourself or, *I did my best.*

Every conversation does not have to be *the* conversation, but the end of life can bring about a sense of urgency to honestly share your love, gratitude, or forgiveness.

There are many ways to share love with others

Write a love letter to your kids, partner, friend, or grandbabies.

Dust off old journals and put them in the hands of someone trustworthy.

Ask someone to try one of the activities in this book with you.

Gift precious items to people. When my daughter was six, she asked, "Mama, can I have that black thing with two drawers when you die?" So, lucky her: she gets the file cabinet.

Sit in silence together.

> Give and receive touch—hugs, hold hands, or whatever feels good to you.

What should I do for myself during this time?

In general, you should do whatever you want to do. Consider the question, What do I really want to do before I die? My mom went to Hawaii the year she died —that was her wish. She dragged her oxygen tank and her bathing suit to Kaanapali. The happiness it brought her and the memories for my dad were priceless. And the sooner you think about this question, the easier it will be for loved ones to help you achieve this.

Specifically, it is helpful to do a little self-reflection. Whether you have been on this planet for two years or 102 years, your life matters and you have made a difference to others. It's helpful to acknowledge this at the end of your life. Look back on your life and marvel at all you have done and the people you have impacted.

My dear friends lost their daughter to cancer when she was only two years old. We all marveled at her courage, her resilience, and her strength while going through chemotherapy. Her parents and siblings have integrated this devastating loss into their lives as they continue to live with deep compassion and awareness that life is short. Though only two years old, she had an enormous impact on all who knew her. I will never forget this special girl and the gifts she bestowed upon us. She is one of the reasons I became a hospice nurse.

Reflect on your life. Pull out old photos and discuss your memories with your friends and family. Shamelessly make a list of all the good you have done. Enlist support from your caregiver. Discuss these questions with your family or friends.

Who are the people who love you and who you've loved?

Whose lives have you touched?

What impact have you had in your jobs or professions?

What makes you feel proud?

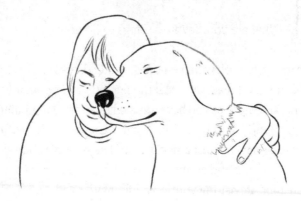

What pets have adored you and have you loved?

What are the values and character traits that make you you?

Which institutions or communities give you a sense of belonging?

What has it been like to raise children? What were you like as a kid?

Do you have spiritual beliefs, and did they change over the years?

> What have been some of the most difficult events that you endured?
>
> What activities have brought you a sense of calm in your life?
>
> What were your favorite things to do as a young person?
>
> What are your favorite things to do now?

Surround yourself with memories, awards, books you love, photos, and memorabilia that reveal the person you are, what you have done, and the lives you have touched. The visual reminders allow your friends, family, and medical team to clearly see you as a whole person, not just a sick person. They may also offer prompts for discussion and soften the emotional intensity of some relationships. Revisiting your own life may provide you with some relief and satisfaction that you lived your life the best you could.

Talking to your family about death

Many patients and families have asked me questions about how to talk to family members, especially children, when facing the potential death of a loved one. Though written with children in mind, much of this advice applies to adults as well.

Be honest and transparent in a gentle way.
People appreciate the truth. Talk directly to them. When children overhear parts of conversations, their imaginations can run wild. Use clear and gentle words like, "Mama has cancer and is dying." Words like passed away or lost or sick are confusing to a child.

They may assume that if Dad catches a cold, he may die too. If they have follow-up questions, answer them sweetly, and simply. It's okay to say, "I don't know." Because often, we can't explain some things, such as why someone gets cancer. Kids may need to hear that it's nobody's fault when someone gets sick.

You don't have to shield your loved ones from your grief. When they see you cry or express your frustration, it normalizes their feelings. Reassure children that they will be taken care of no matter what.

Create memories for later

For those that outlive you, you may want to record video, audio, or written stories about the birth of a child, why their name is so special, advice you want to offer for milestones in their lives, or anything you anticipate wanting to say to them in the future.

Because grief doesn't exactly end, it's important to find ways to integrate this loss into your loved ones' lives gently, softly, and patiently. When thinking about a child, consider what might be beneficial for them as they move through the next many years of their life. What memories might give them strength later? "I remember when you were four years old and you sat next to grandpa when he was at the hospital and you sang his favorite song." Or, "I remember when you were ten years old and you helped mom eat her ice cream when she had cancer. She loved that."

During a visit

Give the child choices: "Do you want to visit Daddy or do you want to draw him a picture?" When a child is visiting a loved one who is dying, I usually say, "You can talk to your grandma. She can still hear you, but she is too tired to talk. You can hold her hand or tell her a story or explain a drawing you made."

Some adults do not like hospitals or anything that has to do with sickness. They will appreciate choices too. They may prefer to video chat, write a letter, or sit in the lobby rather than by the bedside. Everyone has different comfort levels with sickness and some might not even know what their comfort level is yet.

We all grieve uniquely

Grief will come and go and have varying presentations for each individual. Allow the grief to be different for each person, child, or sibling. Kids may want to play, or they may be quiet, and older children or teens may hang with their friends. All emotions are okay: sadness, anger, relief, happiness. Happiness does not betray the person you love. When addressing their feelings, ask children, "What do you think will help you right now? Do you want some time alone? Do you want to sit with me? Do you want to play basketball?" Grief carries big energy—kids may need to play, run, or kick a soccer ball to release this energy. Adults may want to exercise, clean the house, or power wash the deck.

Allow for creative expression

It can be a good idea for both children and adults to have art supplies, crayons, markers, and paper available. Kids (and adults) can't always articulate their feelings at this time. Some hospices have art therapists who can help patients and families find healing through art.

Many hospices offer age-appropriate resources and skilled grief support when you are sick and after you have died. Sometimes your family can meet with these therapists prior to your death to establish a connection. Setting the tone of honesty and vulnerability when talking about death, and giving your family members encouragement to talk about their feelings is a good foundation for beginning to process grief.

Confronting your death may feel overwhelming. Remember to call on friends, family, and professionals. While life review may offer you some space and satisfaction, know that denial is an acceptable place to go also. It is difficult to release our grip on this life that we know and step into the next mystery. But each little step, each tear shed, each morsel of honesty may offer you a release, a softening, and some peace.

A Meditation on Grief

To meditate on grief, let yourself sit alone or with a comforting friend. Take the time to create an atmosphere of support. When you are ready, begin by sensing your breath. Feel the breathing in the area of your chest. This can help you become present to what is within you. Take one hand and hold it gently on your heart as if you were holding a vulnerable human being. You are.

As you continue to breathe, bring to mind the loss or pain you are grieving. Let the story, the images, the feelings come naturally. Hold them gently. Take your time. Let the feelings come layer by layer, a little at a time.

Keep breathing softly, compassionately. Let whatever feelings are there—pain and tears, anger and love, fear and sorrow—come as they will. Touch them gently. Let them unravel out of your body and mind. Make space for any images that arise. Allow the whole story to unwind. Breathe and hold it all with tenderness and compassion. Kindness for it all, for you, and for others.

The grief we carry is part of the grief of the world. Hold it gently. Let it be honored. You do not have to keep it anymore. You can let go into the heart of compassion; you can weep.

Releasing the grief we carry is a long, tear-filled process.

Yet it follows the natural intelligence of the body and heart. Trust it, trust the unfolding. Along with the meditation, some of your grief will want to be written, to be cried out, to be sung, to be danced. Let the timeless wisdom within you carry you through grief to an open heart.

Used with permission from *The Wise Heart* by Jack Kornfield

As You
Are Dying

Chapter 18:
As You Are Dying

Well, dear reader, I will continue to be transparent with you to the end. I trust you will hand your care over to your caregivers when you are ready. Hopefully, you have trained your friends and family along the way and you can soften into this experience, knowing they have the tools and you are not alone.

In the end, this is your death. You can still make choices that reflect who you are and how you would like to exit this world. The next chapter describes what your caregiver can do when you are dying. If your caregivers know what you want, it may eliminate some confusion, which is a lovely gift.

You can now choose to read ahead and insert your requests along the way, or you can simply rest now.

—

Generally, there are two stages of decline before death: transitioning and actively dying, but your age, unique personality, spirit, and body may add some variation or surprises.

> You may have all the signs of dying, and then you may surprise people and rally.
>
> You may have very few signs, and you may suddenly slip out of this world.

> You may die fighting.
>
> You may linger...and keep your family and friends guessing.
>
> You may prefer to die alone.

I have witnessed some families hold vigil for days, and the moment the room is free of other people, the patient shifts and begins actively dying. My guess is, it's difficult to let go of your partner, your friends, or your grandkids—to let go of everything you know—and step into the next mystery. You might want to do it alone, without holding on to anything or anyone.

On the flip side, you may be like my patient Paul who would sweetly grab my hand whenever I was at his bedside. He told me with tears in his eyes, "You know, I thought I would be able to do this on my own. I don't want to. I want you here and I want my family here and I want to hug everyone who comes into my room."

What is transitioning?

Nurses may use the word transitioning to describe your decline as you get closer to actively dying. Though different for everyone, if you are transitioning, you likely have days—or even weeks—to live. If you go through this stage, this is what it may look like.

> You are less responsive.
>
> You may turn inward: you care less about what is going on around you.
>
> You may be less verbal.

You may be physically exhausted and sleeping more each day.

You may eat or drink little if anything.

Patients I've worked with have often used traveling metaphors when they speak, referencing packing for a trip or waiting in lines or boarding a ship. They are preparing for their next journey.

Patients may talk about friends or family members who have died or they may see people who have died. I have been in the room with Jesus and deceased husbands. Patients generally find this experience quite comforting.

What are the signs of actively dying?

Actively dying is when a patient is in the process of *actually* dying. Your body is doing the work of dying. Again, dying is different for everyone, but in general, you may experience some of these physical signs listed and each sign will get more pronounced as you continue to decline. **When these signs are evident, you have hours—or perhaps days—to live**.

You are not verbally responding or actively engaging with the world around you.

You will be sleeping most of the time.

You may appear restless at times. You may reach your hands up into the air and "pick" at nothing.

Your body temperature may fluctuate from hot (sweaty hot) to cool.

You may respond to touch or voice or pain but it is not an active engagement, it is more reactionary.

Your knees and legs and feet may be cool to the touch and will get colder over time.

Your knees will have a very slight blueish/reddish blotchiness called mottling. The mottling will get darker and more pronounced as you are closer to dying.

This mottling will increase and appear at your legs, feet, and the areas of your body that are in contact with the bed.

Your nail beds may appear dusky. Your hands and fingers will get cooler over time. And your arms will also become cool to the touch.

Your wrist (radial) pulses may feel thready or may be difficult to find altogether.

Your urine output will decrease over time.

Your face may appear quite pale or ashen over time. Your nose, your lips, and the area around your mouth may get very pale.

Your breathing pattern may vary a lot.

You may develop a very slight wheezy noise in the back of your throat which may become more pronounced over time. It may remain very quiet or it may get louder over time. This is called the "death rattle" and again, not everyone experiences it. In theory, this should not bother you, it's just fluid moving over your vocal cords.

You may breathe and then not breathe for about twenty seconds, or more, and then breathe again. Your rate and depth of breathing may alternate from rapid and shallow to slow deep breaths to no breathing, like a wave (called Cheyne-Stokes breathing).

When you are very close to dying, your breath may become very shallow, and just the lower part of the jaw moves. Or, you may have significant pauses between breaths, and it appears as though you are opening and closing your mouth without actually breathing. Sometimes a minute can pass between breaths. Or, you may have a gasping quality to your breath (agonal breathing). Or your lips will "puff" out with barely a breath.

You will breathe your last breath.

Your heart will stop.

Being with Dying

To begin the practice, take as comfortable a position as possible, sitting or lying down. Take a few deep soft breaths to let your body settle. Bring your attention to your breath and begin to silently say your chosen phrase in rhythm with the breath. You can also experiment with just having your attention settle in the phrase without using the anchor of the breath. Feel the meaning of what you are saying, without trying or forcing anything. Let the practice carry you along.

May the power of loving kindness sustain me.
May you be happy and free of pain.
May my love of others flow boundlessly.
May all those who suffer be free of pain.
May the experience in some way be a blessing for you.
May I offer my care and presence unconditionally, knowing it
may be met by gratitude, indifference, anger, or anguish.
May I offer love, knowing that I cannot control the course of
life, suffering, or death.
May I find the resources to truly be able to give.
May I remain in peace and let go of expectation.
I care about your pain and suffering, may I be present for it.
I will care for you and I cannot take away your suffering.
May I accept things as they are.
May this experience open me to the true nature of life.
May I see my limits compassionately just as I view the suffering
of others.
May I and all beings live and die in ease.

by Roshi Joan Halifax

Care for the Dying

Chapter 19:

Care for the Dying

L et's now turn our direct attention toward the care-givers. When your loved one cannot direct their own care anymore, your role will shift. Caregivers must take charge through these two final stages in life: transitioning and actively dying.

It is an excruciating honor to be with your loved one when they are dying. I know that your heart is breaking as theirs is slowing. Continue to ask for help. Continue to treat the patient with deep reverence—this is a sacred time.

Here are some ways to support your loved one as they are doing the work of dying.

Call on friends and family. It is difficult to take care of someone who is dying all by yourself. You will need emotional and physical support.

Show up, be present, sit in supportive silence. This is enough. You can send them love and blessings as they are exiting this world. You can read quietly and share space with your loved one.

If you are uncomfortable, take some deep breaths. Inhale. Count to four and release any tension as you exhale, counting to four again. Repeat. Do this any time you feel like you want to leave. It's a compassionate presence exercise—a practice to show up even when you are uncomfortable.

Assume your loved one can still hear and understand you even if they appear unconscious. Friends and family can speak kindly and directly to the patient and discuss events and comings and goings. You can say things like, "Dad, we are going to reposition you now." Or, "Sam is on the phone from Arizona and wants to say hi."

Establish a morning routine. Sometimes it takes days to die. If appropriate, each morning, open the curtains and let some fresh air in. Clean and swab your loved one's mouth, wash their face and hands or bathe them, change their clothes. An easy way to get a shirt on them is to cut the *back* of the shirt from the bottom to *three-quarters* of the way up. If they have hair, brush it every day.

Continue to give critical medications such as scheduled pain meds, nausea meds, or anti-anxiety meds. Ask the hospice team which are the most urgent and critical medications. The patient will likely not be able to swallow safely, so you may have to give them cleverly now in a liquid form or through an oral syringe or rectally. If giving liquids in the mouth, gently and slowly insert into the cheek area or under the tongue.

Clean and moisten their mouth and apply lip balm. Your loved one will not likely be able to safely swallow any longer and their mouth will get dry. Wet the patient's mouth with an oral syringe or a mouth swab, or offer ice chips if they can tolerate it.

Manage their pain and any breathing difficulties. Continue to give their scheduled pain medications. The patient will let those around them know when they are in pain or anxious.

At this time it's your job to take care of them and keep them comfy. Caregivers, look for the typical nonverbal signs of pain, such as grimacing, furrowed brow, gripping, tension in the body, moaning, labored breathing, jaw tension, restlessness, and agitation. If the patient appears to be in pain or short of breath, please call the hospice team for guidance.

Consider the patient's spiritual needs. Would the patient want a priest, chaplain, rabbi, or religious leader to come to their bedside and offer them a final blessing? Your hospice team has a chaplain who may be on call 24/7 and can offer a sacred bedside ritual, or they can find a spiritual leader in your religious community.

Provide ongoing reassurance. Remind them that they are safe, they are home in their bed, and you are with them.

Anticipate pain. If your loved one appears to be in pain with turns, premedicate before you move them. For example, if caregivers are going to turn the patient at 3 p.m., they should administer prescribed pain medication at 2 p.m.

Keep the patient comfy with lots of pillows. If they are lying on their back, you can place pillows underneath their arms or under their knees or under their heels. If they are lying on their side, support their back with some pillows, place one in between their knees and place one in front of the patient's torso to support the top arm. Tuck pillows wherever they may need a little extra cushy support.

Gently reposition your loved one. Caregivers should still reposition (gently move) the patient every two–four hours or so while the caregivers are awake to prevent bedsores. It feels terrible to lie in one spot for a long time. A slight shift of the pillow is better than no movement at all. Move the patient to the right side with pillows supporting them, and then to their back, and then to the left side, and repeat. Some families request their loved ones not be moved at all. This makes a wound care nurse cringe, but when someone is dying, sometimes not moving them is the better, softer choice.

Secretion management. At end-of-life, some patients may develop a slight rattle in the back of their throat. As they are getting closer to dying, this rattle may intensify, but sometimes it doesn't. If the patient has secretions or congestion and it appears to bother them, position the head of the bed upright, or move the patient into a high-side lying position. Certain medications may soften this symptom. Call the hospice team if you have concerns.

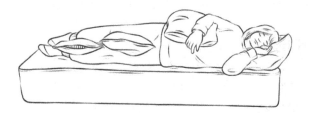

Have tissues available. There will most likely be some tears. I do *not* recommend the recycled tissues for this moment—you want the soft, fluffy, state-of-the-art tissues.

Check their briefs every few hours to make sure they are clean and dry. Sometimes if a patient is nonresponsive and agitated, a wet brief could be the issue.

Wipe their forehead with a moist washcloth if they are hot.

Declare this a laptop-free zone if appropriate. Devices can be distracting. It may help you to consider, "What would I want if I were dying?"

Manage your regrets. What does the patient need to die in peace? What do you need to live in peace? Declarations of love, forgiveness, gratitude? My own dad died suddenly and I still regret that I never told him "thank you" or "I love you" before he died.

Give your permission to go if you feel this is appropriate—you can tell them you love them and it's okay for them to go. I have had a few families refuse to do this as they felt the patient would be insulted. So you have to drop into your heart and do whatever feels like truth to you. There is no right answer—it's only about *your* right answer.

Call up any family or friends if they have any last loving words for the patient. You can hold the phone to the patient's ear.

Go to the bathroom if you need to. If you are concerned about leaving the bedside because you may possibly miss the moment of death, but you desperately have to pee, let the patient know when you will return. I feel like this gives the patient permission to either wait until you return or exit this world when they are ready, which may be when you are not in the room.

Read to the patient from their holy book of choice, poetry, or anything that may bring them comfort.

Laughing and happiness are sacred too. Happiness does not betray the person you love. I think this would be a nice way to exit the world—surrounded by laughter and happiness.

Play music or sing. One of my patient's family members asked for any kind of Elvis music. We found an Elvis Christmas CD and the patient died to Elvis singing Blue Christmas.

Consider the patient's preferences always. Consider *their* religion, *their* values, *their* culture, and *their* philosophies. Some patients want to die to the sounds of their favorite news program, some may value salt lamps, or certain prayers, or Buddhist chanting.

Breathe in, breathe out. I am glad you are there. Sometimes, it's nice to have things to do, to take care of, to consider. I have seen harps and horns, choirs and cuddling, sleeping and soap operas at the end of life. But do know that your presence alone is perfect. Just be. Send them off into the next mystery steeped in love. That is perfect, good work.

The moment of death. What can I do after my loved one has died?

Pause.

Very few moments in life have a definite connection with the divine. This moment is one of them. Take all the time you need: one minute, one hour, seven hours, whatever timeframe feels right to you.

Breathe.

Weep.

Note the time of death.

It is normal to be surprised.

It is normal to feel incredulous.

You can still talk to your loved one.

Witnessing a death can be transformational. You may consider yourself lucky—or not. For some reason, you were part of this extraordinary event.

What if I was not there when my loved one died?

It is important to be kind to yourself if you've missed the moment of death. I have had many experiences in which my patient changed suddenly and began to actively die when the room was finally free and clear of family and friends. I have run out to parking lots in search of their friends who just left, and called every family member at 2 a.m. In spite of these efforts, sometimes the patient dies without family present. Though no one knows for sure, it may be easier for a patient to step into the next mystery without holding on to anyone.

What if I am not comfortable with death or a dead body?

Everyone has different comfort levels with death and dying, and this is okay. If you need help and assistance, please ask friends, family, or your hospice team.

You may not have a choice about when death occurs, but you can do what feels right for yourself after your loved one dies. Some people do not want to be near anyone who has died or may not feel comfortable touching someone who has died. That is okay.

If your loved one has died and you want their body removed as soon as possible, the quick steps are to call the hospice, report the time of death, and ask hospice to call the funeral home. The funeral home will arrive in the next hour or two and transport your loved one's body to the funeral home. If, however, you want to be more ceremonious, this next section is for you.

Suggested care rituals after death

Many cultures have lovely after-death or post-mortem rituals. If you do not have any known rituals and are interested, here are some suggestions.

Respect and honor the patient
I continue to talk to the patient after they have died and treat the patient respectfully as if they were still living.

Bathe or freshen up your loved one
Gather a basin with warm water and soap, and a few washcloths. Reverently clean their body from head to toe. If that feels like too much, you can just freshen up their face and hair. Apply lotion if you wish. Everyone thinks that people lose control of their bowels when they die. Many patients do not, but if it happens, you don't have to clean that up, unless you want to. The funeral home will take care of it if necessary.

Turn off and remove oxygen tubing

Dress the patient
You can fully dress them or keep it simple. Place your loved one
in a gorgeous gown or a favorite shirt. To easily get the shirt on
your loved one, take some scissors and cut up the back. Place
briefs or underpants on—or not. Trust your instincts with this.

Play some music or sing songs
These songs will likely stir memories later on.

Place a beautiful or sentimental blanket over the patient,
keeping the face exposed, if that feels right to you. This blanket
can stay with you afterward and could be a sweet reminder of
your loved one.

Place a flower or two in their hand or on their chest

Light a candle

Freshen the air
I like to quietly but ceremoniously open a window.

**Gather some chairs if you think more people will come
over to visit**

Place fluffy tissues nearby

Consider what rituals were important to your loved one
Is it important to have a priest, rabbi, or chaplain in the room to

offer prayer and ritual? Hospice chaplains are trained to create beautiful rituals. Would poetry, anointing, songs, or prayers be appropriate?

Offer a toast to your loved one
Gather up some pretty glasses and, depending on your family culture, honor your loved one with a sparkling cider or a nice scotch.

Share stories at this time
Everything you do at this time will be part of the memory of your loved one. A ritual may help with your grief and may buoy you during the rough times.

When should I call family and friends to alert them?

Call or text family and friends when you wish. Some may want to visit once more after the death. If they are so inclined, they probably should. I think viewing your loved one after they have died can have a significant impact on your grief process and can help with closure.

When my dad died suddenly of a heart attack, I flew to Southern California the next day. My siblings and I went to the funeral home, and they asked if we would like to see our dad. Oh my, I hesitated. I was terrified, despite being a hospice nurse myself. I walked in and literally fell to my knees. I cried and cried and cried—ugly crying. I released an ocean of tears that day, which helped to soften my pain and eventually process this loss.

When do I call the hospice team?

You can call them right away if you want support. Or you can call them after you have taken time to be with your loved one and feel able to discuss logistics and business matters. The hospice team will contact the funeral home you've chosen, the doctor, pharmacy, and so on—allowing you to focus on family and friends. When you call the hospice, they will want to know:

> The time of death.
>
> If you want them to visit. All team members should be very supportive at this time.
>
> When you would like the funeral home to pick up your loved one. You can suggest the pickup time.
>
> If you need to dispose of any leftover medications. They will offer instructions on the most current and proper way to do this.

When will the funeral home pick up my loved one?

If you have hospice, your hospice team must make the call to the funeral home. The funeral home will arrive at the approximate time that you have requested. If however, your loved one dies at home and you do not have hospice support, you will need to call 911. They will send a first responder to the home to ensure that the death was a natural occurrence, and then the medical examiner will be notified. The first responder will be the one that calls the funeral home.

When the funeral home arrives, they may have a bit of paperwork for you, and information about the next steps. The funeral home will place your loved one in a body bag on a gurney with a quilt. You can request to keep your loved one's face exposed. You can assist with the transfer—or not. They will set a quilt over the body and take the patient out of the home to a minivan. You can ceremoniously walk out with the patient or say goodbye at the threshold—whatever feels right to you. This parting can be painful and difficult. Although I do know one family that played their mom's favorite rock songs and had a dance party out to the minivan.

When my hospice caregiving is over, what do I do next?

My mom did not die dramatically. My sister and I sat beside her and she breathed her last breath. That was it. I waited for the next breath and it never came. I threw myself on top of her and wept like a baby.

I am not normally a dramatic person, but when someone you love dies, all bets are off. Although you have been anticipating it and wondering when it will happen, death still catches you off guard. Grief, loss, despair, and surprise are all normal feelings right now. Relief, happiness, numbness, and fatigue? Also totally normal.

As I held my son's hand and we boarded our flight back home, I was in a daze, wrought with despair, relief, exhaustion. I wondered how all the rest of the world was still living, laughing, eating. Acting like life was normal. Shifting back to my old life (and my new life without my mother in it) took...some...time.

In the immediate hours or days having something to do can help you transition away from caregiving. Consider these suggestions for what to do right now:

> Lie down in the sun and weep, pray, relax, draw, paint, or stretch.
>
> Put on a pot of tea and invite someone over to talk about your loved one's life or death.
>
> Write about the last week in a journal.
>
> Eat a pint of ice cream.
>
> It's okay to wander around confused.
>
> Take a shower. When was the last time you took a shower?
>
> Be so gentle with yourself.
>
> Know in your bones that you did the best you could. And that is perfect. Good work.

I know you don't believe it, but eventually these raw feelings will soften. Or you will regain enough energy to at least brush your teeth again.

Some moments will be better than others, and then some hours will be better than others, and then some days will be better than others. It's important to find some way to integrate this devastating loss, which may be through prayer, one-on-one counseling, support groups, art, etc. Many hospices offer a year of bereavement (grief) support. I recommend trying it when you are ready.

It is a privilege to take care of someone who is dying. The gifts bestowed are many: sweet memories, resilience, unbelievable compassion. Perhaps this experience cracked you open emotionally or spiritually. You are likely a different person than when you started on this journey with your loved one.

Take a moment.

Appreciate your new perspective.

In whatever way feels right to you, thank your loved one who has died—for their memories, for each and every gift you have received from this person and for their life.

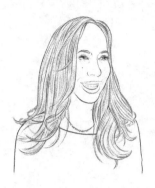

About
the Author

Beth Cavenaugh is a Certified Hospice and Palliative Care RN, with over twenty years of nursing experience. She continues to support terminally ill patients and their families who are in hospice care. Compassion, patient autonomy, and transparent communication are at the core of her care philosophy. She also has a private Reiki practice to support physical, emotional, and spiritual healing for adults and teens.

She lives with her husband in Portland, Oregon, where they have (almost) successfully finished raising their three kids. Her favorite things are lying in the sun, naps, and her spiritual journey.

Acknowledgments

One should never state out loud, "Oh, hey, I'm writing a book," as though it's like emptying the dishwasher. This has been a humbling process. The more I wrote, the more I needed help.

Thanks to the ladies at Works Progress Agency, Emily Fitzgerald and Erica Thomas. Thank you for collaborating on this project and sticking with me as I wandered aimlessly, trying to fulfill a dream I couldn't exactly articulate for months. You are enthusiastic, devoted, and heartfelt people with an awesome eye for art and the desire to change the world one project at a time. Thank you for your guidance, your brilliance, your inspiration, your edits, and consistent encouragement. Since I met you gals, I realize now the possibilities are endless.

Heather-Mariah Violet Dixon, thank you for designing this little beast of a book and turning it into a magical piece of art.

Violet Reed, illustrator extraordinaire. You are so talented, easy-going, and smart. You have a bright future ahead of you. I'm glad I found you early in your career.

I am deeply grateful for my precious family: Kevin, Jack, Grace, and LJ Cavenaugh. Jacko—thank you for deconstructing the book at a critical time. You are all so encouraging, optimistic, loving, and just wonderful human beings. Thank you, thank you, thank you.

Dr. Ben Ware, thank you for your assistance with the clinical details, your multiple edits, and preventing me from misinforming the public. I am humbled by the time you gave, your brain, your genuine presence, and your happy affect.

Ann Eames, thank you for editing my book. A few times. I appreciate your words that were much smarter than mine and your constant encouragement.

Blake Atwood, thanks for your developmental edits, a rework of my work. You kept me focused and clear and reined me in a bit.

Amy Maroney—you are a wonderful friend and a brilliant and funny copy-editor. So lucky to have you in my life and relieved to have your help with this little book.

Anna Gagnon: Chaplain Anna, thank you so much for your thoughtful assistance and insight. Your ability to be present with people is heartfelt and sincere.

Rondi Hunt, MSW, thank you for your input. You are deeply skilled at navigating the big unwieldy issues that arise at end of life.

Dr. Craig Tanner, thank you for your time and wisdom. You have an amazingly present bedside manner infused with lots of humor, which we all certainly value in this line of work.

Kari Morin, thanks for your nutritional contribution to help hospice patients eat healing foods and deep gratitude for your steadfast friendship of a million years.

Jen Bernier, RN, you are one clinically brilliant and deeply compassionate nurse. Thank you for your edits and encouragement.

Sharon Vinhasa, MSW, LCSW. I so appreciate your wisdom and resourcefulness you added to this little book. Thank you for bringing your spirit of aloha to patients living with a terminal illness.

Petya Pohlschneider MSW, LCSW, and Kris Anderson, MSW, LCSW, thank you for your wisdom and insight regarding children and grief.

Kelly Rice, Pharm D., world traveler, adventurer. Thank you for clarifying and simplifying the symptom management information.

Amanda Formosa, RN, Wound Specialist, thank you for your assistance in pressure injury prevention and your thoughtful patient care.

Karen and Mark Wilson, Thank you for the gifts of your friendship, I am inspired by you two every day. Thank you for allowing me to share your very personal story.

Thank you to Ruby Jason (MSN, RN, NEA-BC) for your time, clarifications, and inspiring discussions.

Thank you to Joel Leonard, JD, for your kindness and willingness to guide me through any legal issues.

Thank you to my hospice mentors, teammates, and comrades. I am forever grateful for your wisdom, humor, and compassion.

And of course, thank you to my hospice patients and their friends and families. I honor you and bow to you.

Disclaimer

The contents (text, graphics, images) of this book are for informational purposes only. Though written in good faith, reliance on any information provided by the author is solely at your own risk. I cannot offer a warranty of any kind regarding the accuracy, validity, reliability, or completeness of the information in this book. In fact, it is not even close to a research book. It is written from my instincts, intuition, and experience as a hospice nurse and steeped in my personal and limited perspective on life and death.

This book cannot and does not contain medical advice, and the information provided should never be substituted for real live professional medical advice, treatment, or diagnosis. If you have any questions regarding your medical condition or care, always seek the advice of your physician, hospice team, or other qualified health provider. They know you, your history, and your medical circumstances. If you think you may have a medical emergency, call your doctor, your hospice team, or 911 immediately. Never delay seeking care or medical advice because of anything you have read in this book.

The graphics and images are simply to illustrate my points and provide visual interest. They are not technical drawings and should never be substituted for a medical professional's advice and instruction.

I do share general stories from patients I've had the privilege to care for. To protect their privacy, the patients' names and particular circumstances have been changed.

I do not recommend or endorse any specific tests, physicians, organizations, professionals, products, procedures, opinions, or other information that may be mentioned in this book.

Works Referenced

Asante Hospice Team Members. *Lavender Book: Spiritual Tools for the Dying*. Medford, Or Asante Health System, 2002.

Brach, Tara. "Brief Meditation: Arriving in Mindful Presence." Tara Brach Guided Meditations. July 21, 2016, https://tarabrach.com/brief-meditation-5-minute.

Burn, Jeri. "Overview of Pain Management." Hospice & Palliative Nurses Association, Advancing Expert Care in Serious Illness. 2017. https:/pdfs.semanticscholar.org/755d/cc588f1209f35b02fb-b4045afe610da730b1.pdf.

Byock, Ira. *The Four Things That Matter Most*. New York: Free Press, 2004.

Compassion & Choices. "Understanding Medical Aid in Dying." 2019. https://compassionandchoices.org/end-of-life-planning/learn/understanding-medical-aid-dying/.

Death with Dignity National Center and Death with Dignity Political Fund "Alternative Options to Hasten Death." https:/deathwithdignity.org/options-to-hasten-death.

Death with Dignity National Center and Death with Dignity Political Fund. "How Death with Dignity Laws Work." https://deathwithdignity.org/learn/access.

Dougy Center Staff. *35 Ways to Help a Grieving Child*. The Dougy Center for Grieving Children & Families 2010. 1-42.

End of Life Choices Oregon. "DWD Legal Requirements." https://eolcoregon.org/important-information/legal-requirements.

End of Life Choices Oregon. "End of Life Choices." https://eolcoregon.org/help-end-life-choices-oregon/end-of-life-options.

Halifax, Joan, Barbara M. Dossey, and Cynda H. Rushton. In *Being with Dying: Compassionate End-of-Life-Care Training Guide*. Prajna Mountain Publishers 2007, 82, 187.

Halifax, Joan, Barbara M. Dossey, and Cynda H. Rushton. "Guided Reflective Practice: Boundless Practice for Caregivers." In *Being with Dying: Compassionate End-of-Life-Care Training Guide*. Prajna Mountain Publishers, 2007, 74-75.

Hospice & Palliative Nurses Association. *Core Curriculum for the Hospice and Palliative Registered Nurse*. Edited by Holli Martinez and Patricia Berry, 9-15. Dubuque, Iowa: Kendall Hunt Publishing Company, 2015.

Hospice & Palliative Nurses Association. "HPNA Position Statement–Artificial Nutrition and Hydration in Advanced Illness." HPNA Position Statements. October 2011. https://advancingexpertcare.org/position-statements.

Hospice & Palliative Nurses Association. "HPNA Position Statement–Physician Assisted Death/ Physician Assisted Suicide." HPNA Position Statements. April 2017. https://advancingexpertcare.org/position-statements.

Hospice & Palliative Nurses Association. "HPNA Position Statement–Withholding or Withdrawing Life Sustaining Therapies." HPNA Position Statements. January 2016. https://advancingexpertcare.org/position-statements.

Hospice Foundation of America. "What is Hospice?" https://hospicefoundation.org/Hospice-Care/Hospice-Services.

Kehl, Karen A., and Patricia Berry, In *Core Curriculum for the Hospice and Palliative Registered Nurse*, edited by Holli Martinez and Patricia Berry , 303-317. Dubuque, Iowa: Kendall Hunt Publishing Company, 2015.

Kornfield, Jack. *The Wise Heart: A Guide to the Universal Teachings of Buddhist Psychology, 135.* New York: Bantam Books, 2009.

Kubler Ross, Elizabeth. *On Death and Dying.* New York: Scribner, 1969

Langemo, Diane K. Joyce Black, and the National Pressure Ulcer Advisory Panel. "Pressure Ulcers in Individuals Receiving Palliative Care: A National Pressure Ulcer Advisory Panel White Paper." https://www.woundcarejournal.com 23, no. 2 (February 2010): 59-72.. Lippincott, Williams, and Wilkins.

McDevitt, Amy Z., Margaret Donegan, and Sandra Muchka. "Symptom Management." In *Core Curriculum for the Hospice and Palliative Nurse,* edited by Holli Martinez and Patricia Barry, *99-168. Dubuque, Iowa:* Kendall Hunt Publishing Company 2015.

Naierman, Naomi, and Marsha Nelson. "Choosing a Hospice: 16 Questions to Ask." American Hospice Foundation. 2014. https://americanhospice.org/learning-about-hospice/

choosing-a-hospice-16-questions-to-ask.

National Hospice and Palliative Care Organization "Advance Care Planning." CaringInfo. https:/caringinfo.org/i4a/pages/index.cfm?pageid=3277.

National Hospice and Palliative Care Organization. "Choosing a Quality Hospice for You or Your Loved Ones." Moments of Life. 2014. https:/moments.nhpco.org/sites/default/files/public/moments/Choosing%20a%20Hospice.pdf.

National Hospice and Palliative Care Organization. "Choosing a Quality Hospice for You or Your Loved Ones." CaringInfo. 2017. https://caringinfo.org/files/public/Choosing_Hospice.pdf.

National Hospice and Palliative Care Organization. "Hospice Care." Hospice and Palliative Care. April 3, 2017. https://nhpco.org/about/hospice-care.

National Hospice and Palliative Care Organization *Hospice Care: A Physician's Guide*. Edited by Ann Jackson. Marylhurst, Oregon: Oregon Hospice Association, 2004.

Paice, Judith. "Pain Management." In *Core Curriculum for the Hospice and Palliative Nurse*, edited by Holli Martinez and Patricia Barry, 77-95 Dubuque, Iowa: Kendall Hunt Publishing Company, 2015.

St. Christopher's "Dame Cicely Saunders, Her life and work." https://stchristophers.org.uk/about/damecicelysaunders.

US Dept of Health and Human Services. "What Are Palliative Care and Hospice Care." NIH National Institute on Aging. https://

nia.nih.gov/health/what-are-palliative-care-and-hospice-care.

Winston, Diana. "Body Scan." UCLA's Mindful Awareness Research Center. May 14, 2018. https://uclahealth.org/marc/mindful-meditations.